To Fuse or Not to Fuse

How Artificial Disc Replacement,
Hybrid Fusion, and Fusion
Alternatives are Changing the
World of Spinal Fusion

By
Karsten Ritter-Lang, M.D.
Jan Spiller, M.D.

TABLE OF CONTENTS

DEDICATION

I would like to dedicate this book to my surgical patients, who endured great pain and disruption in their lives prior to deciding to have surgery with me; who shouldered their pain, often in silence, and tried to carry on life while in agony; who learned first-hand how excruciating pain can change one's outlook on everything; who waded through a complex medical system trying to find healing; and who refused to stop at just one doctor's recommendation but performed their own research to find the best possible solution.

I dedicate this book to my patients because they trusted me with their very lives, not simply because I am a surgeon, but because they knew a better life awaited them.

I dedicate this book, as I have my practice and my life, to them.

Karsten Ritter-Lang, M.D.

DISCLAIMER

Some of the information in this book contains anecdotal opinions from the author after practicing extensively and exclusively in the field of spinal surgery and performing over 10,000 spinal surgery procedures and more than 6,500 disc replacements. Unless otherwise stated, statements are based upon his extensive clinical experience of over more than 20 years of practice and are combined with internationally published studies, empirical evidence and a solid scientific foundation.

Medical advice must be modified based upon the patient's individual situation by his/her chosen surgeon and primary care practitioner. The information in this book is intended to serve as a guide to people considering or undergoing spinal surgery. The information presented in this book is in no way intended to replace or contradict any and all information or physician orders set forth by your chosen surgeon or primary care practitioner. All patients undergoing surgery should seek specific advice and recommendations pertinent to their particular situation from their chosen surgeon and primary care practitioner.

INTRODUCTION

WHO IS THIS BOOK FOR?

IF YOU ARE considering undergoing spinal fusion, disc replacement, or another surgical procedure of the spine, this book is for you. Perhaps your physician has told you that lumbar or cervical fusion is your best (or maybe only) treatment option. Or perhaps your pain has become so unbearable that you are seeking treatment options beyond those offered by your doctor. Maybe you have just reached the breaking point where you know you cannot live the rest of your life the way you are now, and *something* must be done. If any of these scenarios apply, this book may be the beginning of a life-changing decision.

What if you have already had back surgery? Perhaps you have a had a discectomy or another spinal surgery and are now feeling the pain and numbness return. Maybe you have had a fusion and are now having additional problems at the levels above or below your fusion site? Or perhaps your doctor has told you it is time to go under the knife again. If so, this book is for you as well.

This book is also for the loved ones of people considering surgery. Perhaps you are a family member, coworker, friend or even a caregiver for someone who has been told they need spinal fusion. You have heard some of the horror stories of those who have had fusion in the past and might be looking for wisdom or a way to provide wise counsel for your loved one. This book is most definitely for you.

IF YOU ARE A DOCTOR...

Lastly, if you are a physician who desires more information about disc replacement and hybrid intervention, presented in a "lay" manner, you, too, may find this book interesting and helpful. Although I have written many scholarly articles and presented to a great number of spine surgeons, this book is written for the ear and eye of the patient rather than the physician. If you are a surgeon and desire more technical information, studies, and more, I would direct you to our website:

http://www.enande.com/resources. There we have compiled a collection of resources just for you.

WHO IS THIS BOOK NOT FOR?

If you have already determined that traditional spinal fusion is your one and only treatment option, and if you are not interested in exploring other options, this book is not for you. If you have been told you require fusion but are unwilling for some reason to seek a second opinion before taking this serious step, this book is not for you.

On the other hand, if you have been previously convinced that traditional fusion is the only way for you, but you are open to learning about cutting edge treatment options that have been shown to help return people to normal function, then read on! You just might find what you are looking for.

HOW TO READ THIS BOOK

People will come to this book from different places. You may be familiar with the architecture of the spine and the types of surgical options commonly available in your home country. Or you may be new to all this and welcome some basic background on the spine and its components before a discussion of the current state-of-the-art in spinal surgery.

For this reason, I have included in Section One a brief tour of the spine and a discussion of degenerative disc disease. This is intended to be a non-technical overview of the spine, the vertebrae and the discs, and is designed to help you better understand my discussion of spinal fusions, disc replacement, and hybrid interventions sometimes referred to as hybrid fusion. Without some understanding of the spine, the differences between these procedures may not be as apparent. But if you are already familiar with degenerative disc disease and the spine as a whole, skip this section and move to Section Two.

Throughout the book, I have intentionally avoided much of the technical language or "medicalese" that most patients encounter. As doctors, we love to be very precise, and there is nothing more precise than the medical terms for procedures, body structures, and functions. But these terms sometimes get in the way of patient-doctor communication. For this reason, I have tried, where possible, to limit myself to common-sense terms and descriptions rather than medical terminology. In doing so, I hope I have made this book easier to read and understand.

Many surgeries, diagnoses, and body parts have more than one name. For example, a disc is also called an intervertebral disc or, intervertebral cartilage. Back fusion is also referred to as spinal fusion, disc fusion, arthrodesis, and interbody fusion. Disc replacement is also known as artificial disc replacement (ADR), total disc replacement (TDR), and intervertebral disc arthroplasty. And a herniated disc is called by many names. Your doctor may choose to use one term over another.

For our purposes, we will be discussing "fusion" rather than "arthrodesis" and will talk about "disc replacement" rather than "intervertebral disc arthroplasty." My hope is that this will make this book more accessible to you and anyone with whom you will share it.

COMPLIMENTARY EVALUATION

You may already know you want to explore disc replacement or hybrid interventions, also sometimes referred to as "hybrid surgery." Or you may know you want a second opinion from me and my highly experienced surgical team. If so, I want to extend to you the opportunity for an in-depth, comprehensive and *complimentary* evaluation. Simply email your full name and email address to evaluation@enande.com, and we will respond right away.

Data from the U.S. Government shows that spinal fusions have increased in the U.S. by 600% in the last 20 years (Whoriskey & Keating, 2013).

WHY I WROTE THIS BOOK

Spinal fusion is a very effective treatment method. When it is appropriate, fusion can turn an extremely painful spinal condition into a relatively painless situation in which load bearing is possible and quality of life is improved.

Spinal fusion is a way to treat several serious spinal problems. But it is not always the <u>best</u> way.

For too many years, and for too many surgeons, spinal fusion has been the "go-to" surgical procedure even when more effective measures were available. This has been true even though spinal fusion has historically been associated with more opiate use, increased disability, and a poor return-to-work outlook (Nguyen, Randolph, Talmage, Succop, & Travis, 2011).

While fusion used to be a surgery of last resort, it is more and more common. In fact, data from the U.S. Government shows that spinal fusions have increased in the U.S. by 600% in the last 20 years (Whoriskey & Keating, 2013).

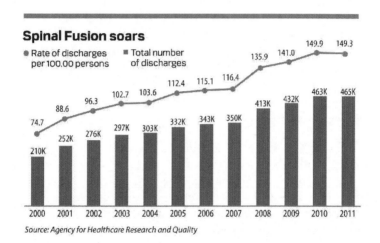

Spinal Fusion soars

- Rate of discharges per 100.00 persons
- Total number of discharges

Source: Agency for Healthcare Research and Quality

In 2011 alone, more than 465,000 fusions were performed in the U.S. according to a study by the Agency for Healthcare Research and Quality. Fusion is actually the most common spinal surgery performed in the U.S. by a very wide margin. Research performed by GlobalData showed that 87% of all the spinal surgeries performed in 2013 in the U.S. involved fusions (Lee, 2014). That is an astounding number.

The growth in the number of fusions has resulted in inquiries about their medical necessity. It has also resulted in accusations that some doctors may be recommending fusion simply for financial gain.

This six-fold rise in spinal fusion is surprising. Or is it? When indicated and properly performed, spinal fusion can be an excellent treatment method. Recent advances in fusion hardware and improved techniques have made fusion more effective than ever. Recovery times and spinal function have improved while

xii

complication and mortality rates have gone down. This is excellent news. Simply put, spinal fusion can be a good solution.

And for many surgeons, fusion is *what they know.* Since other techniques are more recent and some are not yet approved in the U.S. and Canada, surgeons in these countries often go with fusion simply because it is, in their minds at least, the best solution with which they are readily familiar. On the one hand, we can hardly blame them. On the other hand, the extremely steep rise in fusions does make one wonder if there are other motivating factors, especially now that other, often superior, options now exist.

BUT IS FUSION THE BEST SOLUTION?

There are times when fusion is absolutely the best option, but there are far more times when fusion is *not* the best option.

Let me explain.

For many years, people suffering herniated or deteriorated discs had two common options. One option involved a discectomy, where a surgeon removes part of a disc. In this procedure, the surgeon must examine the disc carefully and remove the portion of the disc that is pressing against the nerves in the spine. To gain access and better see the disc, the surgeon may also perform a laminotomy or laminectomy, where part of the vertebra is removed. Discectomy, with or without laminectomy, has been a common solution for many years because it is not as invasive as fusion and has had a lower likelihood of complications.

When a surgeon has determined that discectomy is not appropriate, then fusion has been performed. This involves removal of the damaged disc followed by installation of either a cage or rod-and-screw combination. This hardware helps hold this portion of the spine in a rigid fashion long enough for the vertebra to fuse together, making this once-flexible joint completely solid.

Starting in the 1960's, surgeons experimented with a process to *replace* the damaged disc rather than remove the disc and fuse the joint. Early attempts were unsuccessful. In 1984, surgeons at the Charite University Hospital in Berlin developed the first successful device, the SB-Charite artificial disc, and artificial disc replacement (ADR) was truly born. This is not a discectomy, where part of a deteriorated disc is simply removed.

This is complete replacement of a damaged disc. Hence, it is also sometimes called total disc replacement (or TDR). In the most basic terms, the old, deteriorated disc is taken out, and an artificial disc is put in its place. When performed properly and with the proper artificial disc device, this ADR surgery can be *extremely* effective, even to the point that recipients can experience a return to normal back function and normal activity levels.

In the intervening years, there have been tremendous advances in ADR devices and surgical procedures. Some world-class surgeons have performed thousands of disc replacements. Sadly, despite a great rate of success, very few people have even heard about this incredible procedure. And those who have heard about disc replacement know only a little about it and thirst for information about this surgery. It is for this reason that I wrote this book. For too long have surgeons recommended spinal fusion even when better alternatives exist. The fact that 87% of spinal surgeries in the U.S. involve fusion is astounding. This book is my attempt to elevate awareness of disc replacement surgery and other alternatives to spinal fusion so that you, the reader, can make educated decisions about your own back and the treatment you undergo.

1
THE SPINE

UNDERSTANDING THE SPINE

BEFORE WE CAN talk about spinal disorders and potential surgeries to treat these disorders, it will be helpful to take a quick look at the spine. If you are already familiar with the structure and function of the spine, feel free to skip ahead to the next section.

The human spine gives strength and form to our bodies and is responsible for our ability to stand and walk with an upright posture. It is divided into three sections: cervical, thoracic and lumbar. The spine consists of 24 vertebrae that are connected to one another by intervertebral discs (we will just call them "discs" from this point), facet joints (joints formed from protrusions on the vertebrae) and the various ligaments; together they form a strong but flexible structure. The cervical and lumbar spine are exceptionally mobile. The thoracic spine in conjunction with the ribs forms an almost completely rigid "cage" to ensure the function of the lungs, heart and other organs. In addition to providing strength and structure to the core of the human body, the spine also protects the spinal cord, which runs through the spinal column.

The spine and its components form the major "axis organ" of the body, and all other organs depend on the spine in one way or another. Likewise, the spine can only perform its function with an intact muscular system.

This illustration shows the various sections of the spine in what we call the sagittal profile (seen from the side) and the anterior (or frontal) view. This shows a typical double S-curve, which absorbs loads and distributes or spreads stresses up and down the spine. This curvature of the spine is much like the coil of a spring, which is what allows the spring to compress and still return to its normal form. The same is true of the spine, though to a lesser extent.

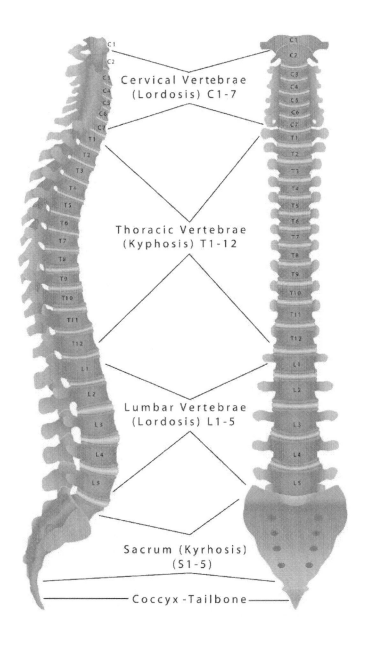

Cervical Vertebrae
(Lordosis) C1-7

Thoracic Vertebrae
(Kyphosis) T1-12

Lumbar Vertebrae
(Lordosis) L1-5

Sacrum (Kyrhosis)
(S1-5)

Coccyx-Tailbone

VERTEBRAE

To understand the disc, you need to first understand the vertebrae. The vertebrae are the bones in your spine. They are what gives strength and structure to your body. Each of the 24 vertebrae in a spine are unique. Though no two are quite the same, they do share common structures and function. The diagram below shows cervical, thoracic, and lumbar vertebra from a top-down view:

CERVICAL VERTEBRA

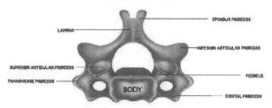

THORACIC VERTEBRA

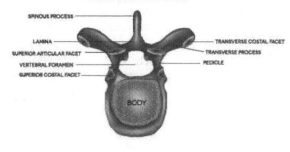

LUMBAR VERTEBRA

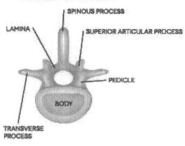

Notice how dramatically the vertebrae change as we move from your neck (cervical vertebrae) down through your mid back (thoracic vertebrae) all the way to your lower back (lumbar vertebrae). The differences, even at a glance, are striking. This is because these vertebrae are formed to behave differently from each other.

The vertebrae in the thoracic spine allow very limited mobility. Instead, with the ribs, they provide a mostly rigid upper core that supports and protects your lungs, heart, and other critical organs. Because of this relatively rigid structure, the thoracic vertebrae tend to bear stresses together, with very limited force borne by an individual vertebra. As such, we see far fewer thoracic spine injuries and degeneration than we do in other areas of the spine.

The cervical and lumbar spine are another story. The vertebrae in a healthy cervical spine and lumbar spine allow significant motion. Barring injury, their form allows you to bend down and touch your toes, and to bend your neck to put your chin on your chest. As you may have experienced if you have back problems yourself, any compromise in motion in these areas can result in serious limitations and pain. The high level of mobility in the lumbar and cervical spine comes at a cost; these areas are far more prone to injury and degeneration than the thoracic spine. The relative freedom of movement means a single lumbar or cervical vertebra can be subjected to much greater stress than a thoracic vertebra. The additional movement also causes these areas of the spine to wear out at an earlier age as a result of degenerative processes. For this reason, lumbar and cervical spine injuries are very common. Unfortunately, because the spinal column also surrounds and protects the spinal cord from injury, changes to the segments of the spine can also impact the spinal nerves structures and cause excruciating pain and other symptoms.

INTERVERTEBRAL DISCS

In between the vertebrae are soft, flexible discs that serve to separate the vertebrae and allow them to move in relation to each other. These are called intervertebral discs for the simple reason that they sit between the vertebrae. For simplicity, they are often referred to merely as discs.

The exterior of each disc is composed of a fibrous material called the annulus fibrosis. This surrounds and protects the soft fluid-filled center, the nucleus pulposus. While the names of these structures are not important, their function is *very* important. You see, this combination of a soft center and a strong but flexible exterior allows the spine to move in six distinct ways.

6 Motions of a Disc

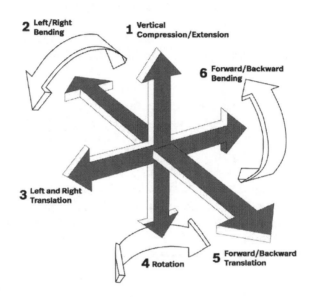

THE SIX DEGREES OF MOTION

1. Flexion and extension (bending forward and backward)
2. Lateral flexion and extension (bending sideways)
3. Rotation (turning or twisting)
4. Forward and backward translation
5. Side-to-side translation
6. Vertical compression

The translation referred to here is the slight amount of slipping motion that occurs when one vertebra moves forward or backward over the disc. Vertical compression refers to the way the discs serve as a cushion between the vertebrae, forming a sort of shock absorber between the them.

These six degrees or qualities of motion create a cumulative flexibility of the spine. No one joint moves very far in any direction by itself. But the combination of many joints each moving a small amount allows us to have significant flexibility in all planes. But all of this depends on the health and elasticity of the discs.

These intervertebral discs are wonderful structures that allow the spine to move in wonderful ways. These discs also help protect the vertebrae from each other, keeping them from wearing against each other. And because of the stresses and motion that these discs must endure for a lifetime, they often get injured as well.

• • •

DEGENERATIVE DISC DISEASE

The structures of the spine are subject to a natural aging process, what we call degeneration. This natural degeneration usually begins shortly after we start growing, around age 18 on average. The symptoms of disc degeneration may begin shortly after this or may not show up until many years later. Many factors can affect degeneration. The aging process is often influenced by genetic factors. Some people are more likely to experience significant degeneration than others, simply based on their genetics. This is why back problems often "run in the family." In addition, this aging process can also be accelerated by external factors. Continuous hard work under adverse conditions, sports injuries and accidents involving great force can accelerate the biological aging processes. All of these factors can lead to significant degeneration of the spine. The boundaries between biological aging and degenerative "wear and tear" are blurred and can lead to spinal problems at any age.

As a result of natural degeneration, back pain is extremely common. Roughly 80% of all people will suffer from back pain sometime in their lives. While this may seem like an incredible number, you likely have encountered enough people with current or previous back pain to know this is correct. Fortunately, only approximately 10% of those affected develop a chronic back pain disorder that creates the need for long-term treatment.

The term Degenerative Disc Disease is a bit of a misnomer. The term actually encompasses a number of processes and disorders that cause a variety of degenerative changes to the discs in the spine. It is not a disease in the sense of something you can "catch" or acquire from an infection. It is, instead, meant to describe a damaged or degenerated state in the disc.

This damage can take many forms. Over time, your discs, which are normally soft and flexible, can leak the fluid that gives them these qualities. As they leak fluid, they tend to shrink and harden, and they lose their ability to flex. The disc can decay and collapse to such a point that it fails to properly separate the vertebrae above and below it.

Your discs may also develop small cracks, tears and fissures over time. As they do, the jelly-like material in the disc can seep out. The disc can eventually disintegrate or break apart, and the remaining portions of the disc can press against the spinal cord.

Sudden disc herniations, where the disc tears and/or portions of the disc contents are pushed outside the normal disc profile, can occur more readily because of degenerative disc disease, and such herniations can also accelerate degenerative disc disease.

Do not think that the "disease" is limited to the discs. This is not the case.

Depending on how advanced the degeneration has become, the motion of the discs and vertebrae will be affected. Over time, damaged discs will shrink. Instability may develop, where the diminished disc allows too much motion to occur.

As a disc shrinks, it also allows the "disc height" to collapse. The disc height is the normal distance between two neighboring vertebrae as they are kept apart by a normal, healthy disc. And a damaged, compressed disc allows the vertebrae to come closer to each other. Sooner or later, this leads to increased contact between the facet joints of the vertebrae, which will, in turn, cause arthrosis, also known as osteoarthritis, and a condition called hypertrophy of the facets.

Now you are probably familiar with the term *atrophy*, where a muscle may get smaller from lack of use or some other condition. Hypertrophy is just the opposite. In this case, it means the facets, having come closer together and more frequently into contact, actually grow *larger*. This can ultimately lead to narrowing of the spinal canal and increased pressure on the spinal cord itself. This complex process can cause great localized and radiating pain, along with numbness, tingling, and more.

In some cases, the vertebrae above and below the collapsed disc may actually fuse to each other, something called an auto fusion.

As discs lose their form, their function in maintaining alignment of the spine suffers as well. The normal curvature of the spine may be disturbed, causing yet more pressure on portions of the spine and impacting its ability to support the body and absorb stresses. Sadly, degeneration in one portion of the spine, subsequently, causes more and more stress and degeneration on other portions of the spine.

As discs collapse or get compressed, the vertebrae above and below may start to form bony fingers or prominences. These are called osteophytes. Over time, these also begin to cause problems, especially when they press against the spinal nerve roots or the spinal cord itself. This condition is called spinal stenosis and can result in extreme pain, numbness, and other symptoms.

All of these conditions are encompassed in the term degenerative disc disease. And, as you can see, while degenerative disc disease is not a "disease" in the way measles is a disease, it is an entire group of problems that develop over time in the discs and surrounding structures of the spine.

● ● ●

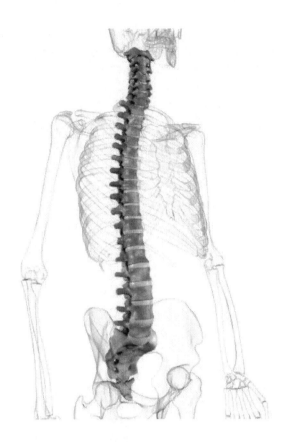

PAIN AND CHRONIC PAIN

SOURCES OF PAIN

Degenerative Disc Disease can cause great pain, and it can arise in a number of different ways.

One of the most common situations we encounter is when the disc is either bulging or torn. In the case of a bulge, the bulge may press against the spinal cord (central bulging) or instead press out to the side (lateral bulging) and compress the nerve roots where they leave the spine. Whenever there is undue pressure against nerve tissue, there is great potential for pain and other symptoms.

This is also true when the outside of the disc, the annulus fibrosis, is torn. This allows a herniation, where the soft interior of the disc is pressed out and against the nearby nerve structures, resulting in pain, numbness, and electrical shock-like feelings. Depending on what nerve structures are compromised, the pain, numbness, or tingling can be localized or instead radiate through one or more extremities.

DISC DEGENERATION

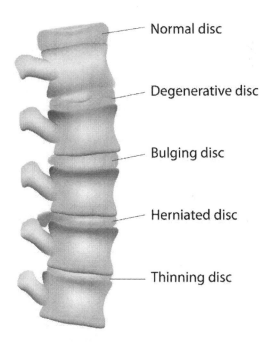

Normal disc

Degenerative disc

Bulging disc

Herniated disc

Thinning disc

Pain can also develop in the rear fiber ring of the disc itself, in the capsules of the facet joints and also in the ligaments and muscles of the back.

The biochemical change of the disc nucleus can also lead to changes in the chemical environment, which will in turn cause pain.

CHRONIC PAIN

Pain receptors along your spine send pain signals to a nerve core area in the brain stem called the pain center. This triggers the pain that you experience. It can also trigger defense mechanisms (fight or flight reflexes). Pain gets very problematic whenever the intensity of the pain signal and the density of the signal leads to a permanent flooding of the pain center. This can lower the threshold of pain and result in a constant perception of pain. This may lead to a pain processing disorder, a completely separate ailment. If pain persists for more than six weeks, it is labeled as chronic pain.

Pain can take many forms. It can be dull, or it can be sharp. It can be a general, widespread sense of irritation, or it can be a stabbing pain. It can be barely noticeable, or it can be excruciating. Pain may also be associated with numbness or a "pins and needles" sensation. Pain can be accompanied by these other symptoms at any stage of the condition. When pain levels and these other factors are present, the quality of life immediately suffers. Even relatively slight or dull pain, if experienced long enough, can impact moods, relationships and productivity. When pain progresses and becomes more severe, basic postures (like sitting or standing) and once easy motions (like walking or bending) can become so painful they can no longer be tolerated. Work and home life can suffer, and depression can set in.

Pain and chronic pain can have devastating effects. For this reason, finding the source or cause of the pain is critical. When the source of the pain can be determined, interventions (surgical and otherwise) may be appropriate.

When attempting to determine a diagnosis of degenerative disc disease, your physician will utilize not just diagnostic films and studies (like x-rays and MRI) but will also want a detailed description of the pain and other symptoms you experience. It is my professional opinion that surgeons should not "treat" MRIs or other indicators. They need to treat the entire patient. MRIs are fantastic tools, but two people with the same MRI findings can have completely different symptoms. The physical problems shown by MRI may manifest very differently across different patients. For this reason, getting a detailed understanding of the pain and other symptoms can be critical to an accurate diagnosis. As you will see below, this is also vital when determining how best to treat these problems.

2

TRADITIONAL TREATMENT OPTIONS

NON-SURGICAL TREATMENT OPTIONS

EXACTLY HOW DEGENERATIVE disc disease is treated depends on a great number of factors. These include the pain the patient experiences, the distribution of the pain, any sensory problems (numbness or tingling), and functional changes (limping, bladder control, decreased reflexes, etc). In addition, treatment may depend on the timeframes in which these symptoms have occurred, the duration and intensity of the symptoms, and more. Your doctor should carefully consider both the qualitative and the quantitative situation then put this information into context with diagnostic results from X-ray studies, MRIs, etc.

The initial treatment for suspected degenerative disc disease is usually conservative in nature. The term "conservative" in medical spheres is usually synonymous with non-invasive or non-surgical measures. Conservative steps such as physical therapy and pain medication are often prescribed to allow the body a chance to heal itself or at least let the symptoms resolve or decrease as much as possible. Other conservative measures can include ultrasound, restricted activities, heat and/or ice, stretching, and more. Conservative care can allow the symptoms of degenerative disc disease to be alleviated without actually removing the cause of the difficulties. Conservative steps can also allow weakened back muscles, often the source of back pain, to be strengthened. While patients sometimes chafe at being told repeatedly that rest, exercises, and pain medication are the best method of treatment, the truth is that many back injuries and spine problems can be cured or alleviated with these measures. There are also a significant number of back injuries that simply resolve by themselves over time.

If you are having back pain, you and your physician should always be very slow to consider spine surgery, except in rare, emergency situations. There are times when spinal fusion is required on an emergency basis because of a critical or catastrophic injury. In these circumstances, surgical decisions may have to be made in days or even hours. In most cases, however, surgery should only be considered when non-surgical treatments have been tried and found ineffective. Thorough conservative therapy usually means at least six months of consistent pain management through medication and physical therapy. While you will read later in this book about the extremely positive outcomes we have had with disc replacement, even this very successful procedure should be performed only if conservative care has been exhausted first. Surgery has risks associated with it, and you should not undergo such risks unless you absolutely need to.

SURGICAL TREATMENT OPTIONS

If the structure of the spine has become too damaged to respond to non-surgical measures, other, more-invasive steps need to be considered. If a patient demonstrates chronic pain, poor spinal function, and compromised quality of life, we must consider surgical options.

There are several types of surgeries that can be used for patients with degenerative disc disease. While spinal fusion is *by far* the most common spine procedure performed in the U.S., and perhaps in Canada as well, it is only one of many options. Which one is right for you depends on your diagnosis along with many other factors.

Spinal procedures are often divided into two different categories. These are Symptomatic (meaning the surgery is performed to address the symptoms of a disease without addressing the underlying pathology) and Reconstructive (where the actual structure of the spine is repaired or corrected).

SYMPTOMATIC SPINAL PROCEDURES:

Here is a list of what we would categorize as Symptomatic back surgeries:

Intradiscal Electrothermal Therapy (IDET): IDET involves the controlled application of heat to the disc through a thin wire. The general theory is that the heat will cause contraction of the disc and some thickening of the exterior of the disc, possibly narrowing or closing fissures on the disc. While this can be performed micro-invasively, the benefits are questionable.

Laser Discectomy: Several methods of using lasers to treat spinal conditions have been attempted. The outcomes have thus far fallen short of expectations. The general idea is that a surgeon will direct the laser onto tissues impacting the nerve roots and destroy these tissues with the concentrated heat of the laser. Thus far, the end result has not been superior to more traditional methods of accomplishing the same task, at least in regards to the spine.

HydroGel: One of the simplest and least-invasive of spinal surgeries is relatively new and involves injecting a disc with "HydroGel." This fluid is intended to replace the fluid that has leaked out of a damaged disc. This very quick procedure can restore reasonable function to a damaged disc at least for a time. Unfortunately, this procedure cannot be performed if the disc is substantially degenerated since the fluid will not be contained in the disc. Furthermore, the benefits of injecting HydroGel are limited in duration and will vary depending on numerous factors, the condition of the existing disc being the most important.

Endoscopic Treatments: This refers to a Symptomatic surgery accomplished with endoscopy, using a small camera or scope to work on the spine through a small opening. Such a method can be utilized to carry out a wide variety of procedures

Microdiscectomy: This minimally invasive surgery requires incisions as small as one inch. Using specialized tools and magnification, the surgeon removes one or more spinal fragments from the spinal canal. The idea is to remove the portion of the disc material that is causing problems while leaving the rest of the damaged disc in place. This surgery can often be performed on an outpatient basis. Where hospitalization is required, it is much more brief than the hospital stays associated with traditional discectomy.

Discectomy: Many spinal procedures involve partial or full discectomy (also called discotomy), where a portion or all of the disc is removed. This is often employed when a part of the disc has torn off or has been pushed against the nerve root or spinal canal. Other procedures may involve removal of bony fingers or spurs that can develop on the vertebrae and/or widening of the spinal call when it has been compromised. The unfortunate part about most of these procedures is they are temporary fixes to a long-term problem. Removing the bone spurs does not remove the cause of these spurs; over time, the spurs are likely to develop again. Removing all or part of a disc does not repair that disc or restore the proper function of the disc. These procedures simply remove some of the sources of spinal pain but leave the spine prone to recurring problems. In fact, in my experience, roughly half of the patients who received such symptomatic procedures return for surgical intervention at the same level within 10 years. Several medical studies show this alarming statistic as well. This is not good.

Foraminotomy or Foraminectomy: The nerve roots exit the spine through passages called the foramen. Conditions like facet arthritis, disc herniations, and spinal stenosis can narrow this foramen, placing pressure on the nerve root. This is a common source of radiating pain and numbness. These conditions can be treated by widening the foramen, usually by removing soft tissue and bone from this channel. This is called both foraminotomy and foraminectomy. The terms are largely interchangeable, though foraminectomy often refers more appropriately to the removal of large amounts of bone and tissue. This type of procedure is often performed in association with other spinal surgeries, including discectomy/discotomy, disc replacement, laminectomy, and spinal decompression. This is also performed frequently with spinal fusion.

Laminectomy or Laminotomy: One way to treat the narrowing of the spinal canal is to remove a portion of the vertebra called the lamina. This opens of the space for the nerve roots and spinal cord, removing pressure from impacted structures.   The lamina is reduced in small portions using specialized tools until the proper size is reached.

Kyphoplasty or Vertebroplasty: A relatively new procedure, this involves using bone cement to help support a damaged vertebra. This can be used to treat fractures of the vertebra that have occurred because of osteoporosis, trauma or tumor.

A comment about Symptomatic Surgery:

Symptomatic surgery is called this because it addresses the *symptoms* the patient is experiencing without addressing the underlying cause or process that is the source of the symptoms. Such surgeries are often little more than band aids (albeit very expensive and painful band aids) to help reduce pain for a limited amount of time. Some of these procedures may give relief for only a year or two. Others, for 10 years or more. Medical studies show that about 50% of the people who undergo these Symptomatic surgeries (discectomies/microdiscectomies, laminectomies, foraminotomy, IDET, laser, etc) must have further surgery *at the same level* within 10 years. Many require additional surgery in a much shorter period of time. Some unfortunate patients undergo Symptomatic surgery only to discover that emergency fusion is immediately required. For these reasons, exploring the proper reconstructive options is often a better solution.

RECONSTRUCTIVE SPINAL PROCEDURES:

Laminoplasty: One method of treating the narrowing of the spinal canal in the cervical spine is laminoplasty. This requires the lamina to be split apart. Laminoplasty is usually performed across more than one level of the spine as an alternative to cervical fusion.

Spinal Osteotomy: Osteotomy is the term to describe the controlled breaking or cutting of bone. During some spinal procedures, this is necessary to decompress a nerve or install hardware. On some occasions, bone must be cut to realign the spine, and then hardware must be installed to maintain the correct position of the spine. Many methods have been developed to carry out osteotomy where needed. The main goal of this intervention is to improve the sagittal balance.

Thoracoscopic Release: This refers to a correction of a portion of the thoracic spine accomplished through endoscopy, using a tiny camera or scope to work on the spine through a small opening. Such a release involves removing all or part of discs, separation of ligaments, and sometimes the removal of a portion of one or more ribs. This is sometimes performed in conjunction with a Posterior Thoracic Fusion.

Spinal Fusion: Fusion involves physically restraining the motion of the degenerated disc through a variety of methods and approaches. Regardless of the approach, fusion usually requires the surgeon to remove the degenerated disc, install a cage, and then pack the caged disc space with appropriate filling material. This material may come from the patient (from a separate surgical site-often the iliac crest) or from cadaver bone. Other graft materials, including some derived from coral, are used at times. Once the graft material is in place, the surrounding vertebrae are connected with rods and screws. The hardware must then hold the vertebrae rigidly in place long enough for the graft material to fuse to the vertebrae. This can take six to nine months or more. The hardware is usually left in place permanently.

FUSION: A NONFUNCTIONAL SOLUTION

We call fusion a "nonfunctional" solution because it removes the normal function of the disc (motion and shock absorption) and replaces this with rigidity. In fusing the vertebrae together, the proper disc space can be restored and pressure removed from nerve roots and the spinal cord. For this reason, this solution can be quite effective. It can restore a certain quality of life by removing pain and other symptoms. It is also very permanent. Once fused, barring some severe accident or disease, the vertebrae will always be fused. Unfortunately, this also means that the lack of motion and shock absorption associated with a healthy joint are also *permanently* removed.

Fusion has become the preferred procedure for spinal surgeons across North America. In fact, fusion has become so prevalent that 87% of spine surgeries performed in the U.S. in 2013 involved fusion (Lee, 2014). This is an astounding statistic, especially since fusion used to be the surgery of last resort. Now, for many surgeons, a recommendation for fusion seems almost automatic.

SIDE EFFECTS OF FUSION

Unfortunately, fusion, while common, is not without side effects. First and foremost is motion loss in the fused portion of the spine. The combination of spinal fusion hardware and the fused vertebrae themselves leaves this portion of the spine, by design, devoid of any motion in any plane. Where the healthy joint moves in six different ways, the fused joint is completely rigid. This loss of motion causes its own set of problems and has created an entirely new disease, *Adjacent Segment Disease*, as you will see below.

Depending on the type of procedure the patient has had, the hardware placed in and around the spine may also become a source of pain later in life. The hardware can sometimes move over time. This is called implant migration. Such motion can render the hardware ineffective and may require a second surgery to remove or replace the hardware.

Hardware can not only move, but it can also break. In such circumstances, the hardware may come into contact with structures (nerves, blood vessels, joints etc) and cause difficulties. Fortunately, so-called "hardware fracture" is unlikely in most surgeries.

Another potential long-term complication with spinal fusion is pseudo-arthrosis. This means "false joint." Sometimes a fusion just does not work. Despite implantation of hardware and bone material, the vertebrae may not actually fuse. This may allow motion between the vertebrae when the surgeon was trying to eliminate motion. In such a state, the spine pain that necessitated the surgery may continue or even worsen. This "false joint" may also place stress on the fusion hardware, cause it to bend, tear, or fracture. The surgeon may be able to address pseudo-arthrosis by replacing hardware, packing more bone material into the joint, or implanting an electronic device to attempt to stimulate fusion. While long-term pseudo-arthrosis is rare, there are some cases where fusion ultimately fails to ever occur.

ADJACENT SEGMENT DISEASE

For years, we have known that fusion at one level of the spine causes challenges at adjacent levels. When we fuse two or more vertebrae together, we leave the surrounding portions of the spine to "take up the slack" in providing the motion and shock absorption functions of the spine. The additional stresses placed on adjacent discs and vertebrae can cause increased disc degeneration at those levels. This has become so common now that it has been given the name Adjacent Segment Disease and encompasses a number of complications and problems that arise in the areas of the spine immediately above and below the site of a spinal fusion. In my experience, approximately 15% of patients who have spinal fusion require surgical intervention at adjacent levels within the following 10 years. One recent study has found that 22% of patients with lumbar fusions require surgery at adjacent levels within the next 10 years (Sears, et al., 2011). For many patients, a greater than 20% chance of another back surgery within 10 years is unsatisfactory.

> *When we fuse two or more vertebrae together, we leave the surrounding portions of the spine to "take up the slack"*

When properly performed, disc replacement largely eliminates the chance that a patient will develop Adjacent Segment Disease. The natural motion afforded by a device like the M6 Artificial Disc helps stresses and shock absorption to be distributed evenly up and down the spine and avoids the extra pressures and degeneration caused by fusions. To put it plainly, the implantation of an artificial disc at one level does *not* increase the likelihood of surgical intervention at adjacent levels. In fact, instead of 22% of fusion recipients needing attention for adjacent levels within 10 years, *only 2%* of those with disc replacements need surgical intervention at adjacent levels within the same time period. Looking at this statistic differently, those who have fusion are 10 times more likely to need surgery at an adjacent level than those who have disc replacement.

> *Those who have fusion are 10 times more likely to need surgery at an adjacent level than those who have disc replacement.*

The sad part is Adjacent Segment Disease does not stop at just the adjacent segments. Someone who has an initial fusion at one level and requires subsequent fusion at the level above that fusion is now more prone to develop problems at the level adjacent to the new fusion. In this fashion, Adjacent Segment Disease at one level can require fusion at that level and cause Adjacent Segment Disease at the next level. It is therefore conceivable that a fusion at one level can lead ultimately to fusions at many levels over time. This is particularly troubling when we see young, otherwise active patients undergo fusion because they are even more likely to experience this cascading need for additional fusions.

Despite the prevalence of Adjacent Segment Disease following fusion, spinal fusion continues to be the preferred surgical procedure in North America. When we think about it, this should not be surprising. Surgeons and their patients want permanent solutions, and fusion has been the only permanent solution available in the U.S. and Canada for many decades. With the development of disc replacement options, however, we now have another method to permanently treat patients with degenerative disc disease. While disc replacement is available in only a limited way and with limited hardware options in North America, it has become a widely preferred treatment method in other portions of the world, where it has been employed in tens of thousands of cases for more than 30 years.

FAILED BACK SYNDROME

One of the most frightening possible outcomes of spinal fusion (and many other spinal surgeries) is a condition called failed back syndrome. This can result when someone completes one or more spinal surgeries but continues to have dramatic, chronic pain. Sometimes this occurs when people have *more* pain following surgery. Failed back syndrome can be associated with continuing spinal disc herniation, continued pressure on spinal nerves, hypermobility of joints in the spine, development of scar tissue, and more. Sadly, it is often accompanied by anxiety and depression.

Unfortunately, when a patient reaches this point, having had one or more unsuccessful surgeries, additional surgery may no longer be an option. The chronic nature of the pain and lack of improvement from the prior surgeries may signal to the doctor a less-than-favorable outcome for any additional surgery.

Treatment options in such cases are usually limited to pain management, long-term medications, and other conservative measures. The chronic pain and long-term medication intake sometimes lead to the installation of a morphine pump, a last resort for management of pain.

One of the few surgical options sometimes used to treat failed back syndrome is Artificial Disc Replacement.

One of the few surgical options sometimes used to treat failed back syndrome is Artificial Disc Replacement. Such a recommendation must be made carefully and only after addressing all the factors associated with failed back syndrome. The likelihood for a successful surgery at this point is usually less than if Artifical Disc Replacement had been carried out initially.

CASE STUDY: CURTIS SMITH

3-level lumbar artificial disc recipient, with surgery performed in 2014:

I am an administrator at an elementary school in Central California. I have two kids and a wonderful wife, and they are so glad about my surgery!

I blew my back out in 2013. I was moving some wood around my yard when I heard three loud pops in my low back. That started a year of suffering for me. I started having pain and numbness, and it got worse over time. It became too painful to stand or even sit for more than a few minutes, and I ultimately had to take leave from work. I spent most of the next year living on the floor in our home. It was too painful to sit with my family for dinner, so I ate from the floor next to the table. I couldn't sleep in a bed (even with a board in it), so I slept on a thin mattress on the floor. And as my desperation became worse, I began to research solutions from the floor too.

My doctors in the U.S. told me I needed three- or four-level fusion. At age 41, I knew that these fusions would not likely be my last since the adjacent levels would probably need fusion too sometime later. I am an active guy. I play water polo, knee board, and I love to play and wrestle with my kids. My doctors told me I would have to have fusion and then change the way I live to protect my fusion and delay the need for more fusions. I couldn't imagine spending the rest of my life this way. So I researched my options.

Fortunately, my brother-in-law knew a man who received two artificial discs in Germany many years before. He connected us, and my eyes were opened to the possibility of total disc replacement. I saw the long-term result he had and I knew I needed to learn more.

CASE STUDY: CURTIS SMITH (CONT.)

I spent the next several months researching disc replacement through my doctors and the internet. One of my U.S. surgeons offered disc replacement, but he told me he could do so at only one level, and with a device that was less than ideal (though approved for use by the FDA). The more I looked, the more evidence pointed me to the M6 disc by Spinal Kinetics and the surgical team of Dr. Ritter-Lang and Enande. That the M6 was right for me was clear. It was the only disc I encountered that replicated all six motions of a normal disc, even compression. Though it is made in the U.S. only a few hours from my home, I learned I would have to travel out of the U.S. to get it. And this is where Enande and Dr. Ritter-Lang came in. Dr. Ritter-Lang had done the disc replacement for my brother-in-law's friend, and this man had referred many other people to Dr. Ritter-Lang with excellent results. After doing countless hours of research and checking all my options, I chose to have Enande and Dr. Ritter-Lang treat me.

I underwent a 3-level lumbar disc replacement in May of 2014. Although the first week of recovery was tough, they took excellent care of me. Upon discharge from the hospital, they transferred me to the Park Hotel. What a beautiful hotel! And in the midst of a gorgeous park. It was the perfect place to walk and recuperate. I even rode a bike some! On my return home, I was finally able to get back to work full-time and without any medication. More importantly, I was able to eat with my family at the table and be the kind of father and husband God intended me to be!

My back gets tired and sore sometimes, but this is nothing like the agony I had before. The soreness goes away if I stretch and rest a little. Even more, I can do things once again. I have returned to knee boarding, sledding, water polo, snow skiing and all the other things that make up my life. And I can play and wrestle with my kids again!

This is a miracle to me. So praise the Lord! And I will always be grateful for Enande, Dr. Ritter-Lang, and the entire surgical team.

Curtis Smith, Clovis CA USA

3
FUSION ALTERNATIVES

ARTIFICIAL DISC REPLACEMENT

OFTEN REFERRED TO as "ADR," artificial disc replacement (or simply disc replacement) involves removing a damaged or compromised disc in the lumbar or cervical spine and replacing it with an artificial disc, a specially-designed implant created to mimic the natural function of the disc.

By inserting the artificial disc into the spine in place of a damaged or deteriorated disc, the normal movements and strength of the spine can be restored. Restoring normal motion and strength at the level of the artificial disc also assists discs at the levels above and below the artificial disc by alleviating any additional strain caused by a deteriorated disc, or a fusion designed to treat a deteriorated disc.

I have asked Dr. Jan Spiller, Chief Surgeon at Stenum Hospital, to describe this process in more detail.

DISC REPLACEMENT PROCEDURE

Let me describe a disc replacement surgery for you, using as an example a lumbar disc replacement procedure. The cervical variation of the surgery is extremely similar, so much of what I share here applies to cervical procedures as well. To make this easier to understand, I want to include some illustrations of disc replacement using the M6 artificial disc from Spinal Kinetics:

First, our surgical team has found that lumbar disc replacement is best accomplished using what is called an anterior retroperitoneal approach. This simply means we go in from the front of the abdomen and work around and behind the peritoneum or intestinal sac. By staying outside the intestinal sac, we have to pierce fewer membranes, which means fewer sutures and lower potential for complications. We begin with a small incision below and somewhat to the left of the navel or belly button. This incision is considered "minimally-invasive" because the incision is usually shorter than 10 cm (under 4 inches) in length. We work our way around the intestinal sac; there is no need to cut or separate any significant blood vessels, nerves, or organs. Shortly thereafter, we can clearly see the front (or anterior) portion of the lumbar spine.

Using specially-engineered instruments, the existing, damaged disc is removed in its entirety. This includes removing any torn or separated portions of the degenerated disc and especially those portions that are pushing up against the nerve roots or spinal cord. While there, we perform a spinal channel decompression. We remove any bone growth or bone spurs that have grown into the spinal channel. This creates a clean surface for the spinal implant and removes the source of much pain in the spine.

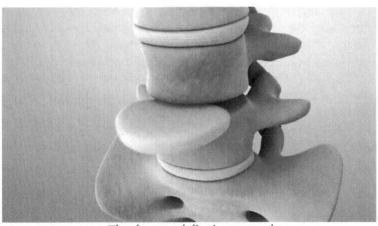

The damaged disc is removed

Next, we use a measuring tool, slipped between the vertebrae, in order to determine the proper footprint for the M6. The device is available with several different footprint sizes. Determining the proper one is very important.

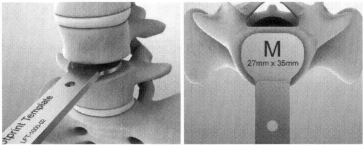

The proper footprint is determined

Next, with the damaged disc out the way, the original disc height is restored utilizing special instruments designed for this precise purpose. Restoring the natural disc spacing relieves a great deal of pressure on the surrounding structures.

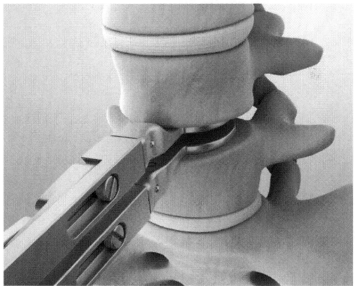

Using special tools, the original disc height is restored

We then carefully measure the vertebrae and disc spaces to determine the proper height and angle (lordosis) of the artificial disc. Fortunately, the M6 devices come in several sizes, heights and angles so a perfect match can be found.

Using special tools, a temporary disc of the proper footprint, height, and angle is placed between the vertebrae as a sort of placeholder or marker. We then use a portable x-ray machine to take intra-operative x-rays of the spine and the temporary disc in order to make sure we will have the best location and alignment when we implant the permanent disc. Once we have verified (and only when we have verified) that the temporary disc is in the proper location, we proceed to the next step.

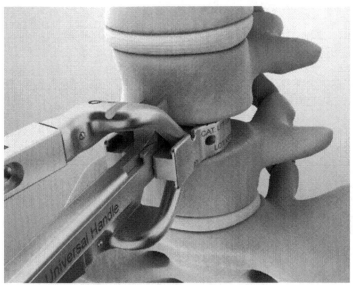

A temporary disc/spacer is installed

We next prepare the vertebrae surfaces to receive the artificial disc. A special tool is used to cut channels in the vertebrae. The channels hold the "keels" of the artificial disc and help it to stay in place.

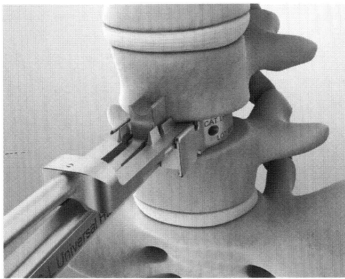

Channels are cut in the surrounding vertebrae.

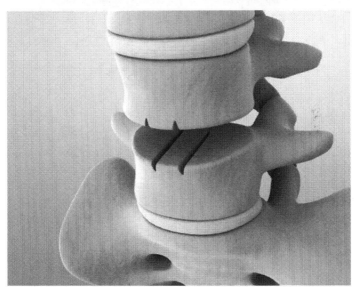

The intervertebral space, ready to accept the artificial disc

With the surrounding vertebra properly prepared to accept the disc, the disc is then pushed into place. The serrated keels of the disc will line up perfectly with the channels previously cut by the surgeon. These channels guide the disc into place, and the serrated shape of the keels will help to immediately hold the disc in place between the two vertebrae.

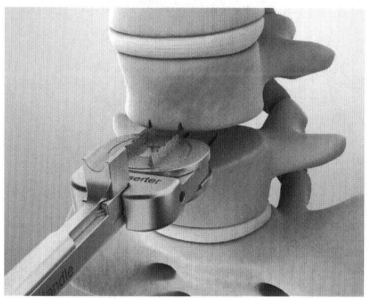

Inserting the artificial disc.
Note the serrated shape of the keels.

With the artificial disc in place, another intra-operative x-ray is taken from several angles to verify the artificial disc is perfectly located in the spine. The new disc will mate perfectly with the vertebrae above and below it. In fact, the new disc and the vertebrae above and below it fit so well together that no cement, screws, or other devices are needed. This initial or primary stability (as we call it) is so stable, the patient will be able to get up and move around in the next 12-24 hours without fear of any movement or migration of the artificial disc. The top and bottom surfaces of the disc are also coated with a titanium plasma spray to promote bone ingrowth and fusion between the disc and the surrounding vertebrae. Ultimate stability occurs within 6 weeks.

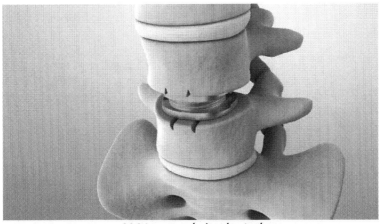

M6-L properly implanted

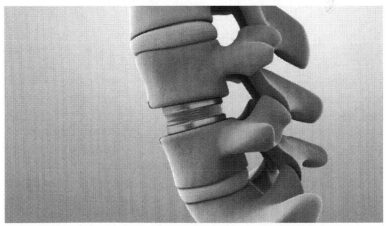

Side or lateral view of a properly implanted M6-L device.

Once we are satisfied with the result, then we can begin closing the surgical site or instead move on to replace another adjacent disc if indicated.

From start to finish, single-level disc replacement surgery usually takes our team about an hour, and multi-level disc replacement is usually accomplished in 60 to 90 minutes. These procedures can be done in a very efficient manner because of the number of surgeries we have performed together as a team and due to the fact that we perform disc replacements many times a week on average. Because the surgery is short, the patient is under anesthesia for only a short time. In addition, due to the minimally invasive manner in which we perform the surgery, blood loss is very minimal, usually less than seven ounces.

While disc replacements have advanced over time, nearly all implants lacked another critical function of the disc: shock absorption.

Cervical disc replacement is very similar. The greatest difference is the nature of the approach. We enter through a small incision in the neck, to one side of the esophagus. We are able to work around this and other structures to visualize the front (or anterior) portion the spine. The preparation and execution of the disc implantation is essentially the same, except with somewhat different tools and much smaller artificial discs.

--Dr. Jan Spiller, Stenum Hospital Chief Surgeon

DISC IMPLANT AND DESIGN

The design of the implants themselves varies significantly and has for years; initial efforts at disc replacement involved borrowing successful technology from knee and hip replacements in an effort to incorporate them into spinal treatment. Surgeons had been replacing knee and hip joints for many years, so such methods were taken and employed for the spine. The initial results were promising but imperfect. Early artificial discs involved a ball-and-socket style joint. While this is a perfect type of joint for a hip, it is not the perfect solution for the spine. Early artificial discs (and even some current ones used in North America today) allowed *too much* motion, more than a natural disc allowed. This additional motion had the potential effect of placing more pressure and strain on surrounding tissues and structures. Early discs also tended to "migrate" or move out of optimal position. This caused several challenges and, in time, required removal or replacement of the implant. Lastly, while disc replacements have advanced over time, nearly all implants lacked another critical function of the disc: shock absorption.

The spine is, among other things, like a large shock absorber that allows us to move, run, and jump without sustaining injury. The spine accomplishes this through a combination of curvature of the spine and the compressible nature of the discs. Each disc in your spine can compress a small amount. Multiply this amount across all the discs, and you have a very effective shock absorber for the body.   The early artificial discs could not compress at all, so they lacked this important function.

Over the years, several generations of artificial discs have been developed. The latest and most effective ones restore the proper amount of motion to the spine and provide an amount of compression or shock absorption similar to a natural disc. The first disc to effectively incorporate shock absorption is the M6 disc from U.S.-based Spinal Kinetics. Unlike other implants, the M6 allows motion in all planes, but in a way that is limited like the natural disc.   It allows forward, backward, and side-to-side bending. It also allows twisting. But the limited compression of the disc makes this disc the first to truly replicate a normal disc. Because it is constructed from a combination of rigid and flexible materials, it provides a level of shock absorption very similar to a natural disc.

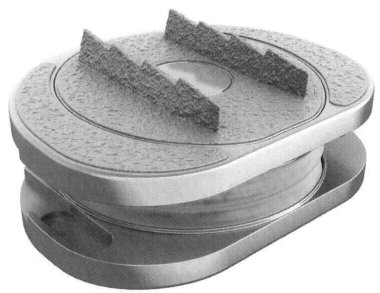

The M6 from Spinal Kinetics

Only with the M6 prosthesis, which we have been using in the cervical spine since 2005 and in the lumbar spine since 2009, has a prosthesis become available that can biomechanically mimic the natural disc. In addition, the M6 prosthesis has been thoroughly investigated biomechanically and has shown very high durability in testing. The M6 prosthesis can complete 30 *million* cycles of motion without exhibiting any significant wear or damage. This means the prosthesis will likely last *at least* 60 to 75 years before suffering wear. This is far superior to the wear cycle of the human disc. For this reason, the M6 disc is preferred around the world by spinal surgery teams that specialize in artificial disc replacement. In fact, as of the writing of this book, over 43,000 M6 discs have been implanted worldwide.

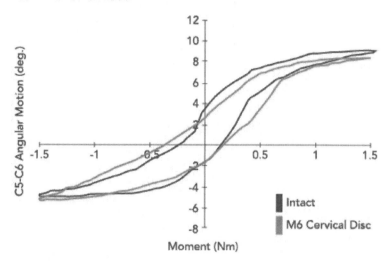

C5–C6 Flexion-Extension Load-Displacement Curves
150 N Follower Load

The illustration above shows how loads are displaced in a natural disc and how closely the M6 disc replicates these load displacements.

Artificial disc replacement has now been shown to be far superior to traditional fusion for the vast majority of patients with degenerative disc disease.   While fusion is sometimes still indicated, many spinal fusions can be avoided through effective artificial disc replacement, and usually with far superior results. In addition, disc replacements at multiple levels are quite common and can be performed without increased complications. While there is a common understanding among many people that more fused levels equal more problems, the same is not true for artificial disc replacement. If the proper implant is used, the artificial disc mimics the natural disc. Therefore, the presence of multiple artificial discs does not increase the likelihood of short or long-term complications. Many patients, rather than undergo a multiple-level fusion, will have multi-level disc replacement. Where indicated, two-, three- and four-level disc replacement can be accomplished in *one* surgery and with excellent results. While it is rare that we would implant four artificial discs, it can and *has* been done with superb results. In fact, we find that the complication rate for multi-level interventions is roughly the same as for single-level interventions.

Where indicated, two-, three- and four-level disc replacement can be accomplished in one surgery and with excellent results.

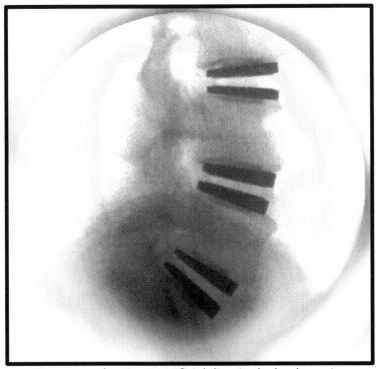

Bone scan showing 3 artificial discs in the lumbar spine

Surgery times for fusion vary depending upon the nature of the procedure and the skill of the surgical team, but a timeframe of two to three hours is not uncommon. The typical ADR surgery performed by our team takes less than 75 minutes. The effects of this are profound. Less time on the table means less time under anesthesia. Less time under anesthesia greatly decreases the likelihood of any complications related to anesthesia. A shorter period of time in surgery also decreases blood loss and the trauma normally associated with surgery. In addition, the anterior (frontal) approach used for disc replacement causes far less trauma than a posterior (from behind) approach used for many fusions. This anterior approach, therefore, results in much faster recovery from surgery as well.

Keep in mind, the ADR surgery durations quoted above are from *our* team. We have a team of surgeons and support staff used to performing ADR surgery on a frequent basis. In fact, we perform ADR surgery more than 250 times a year, and we have performed thousands of such surgeries. Other surgeons may not enjoy the advantages of such an experienced team. Some surgeons who perform ADR surgery do so a handful of times a year. There are days where our team performs that many ADR procedures *in a day*. This makes a substantial difference in surgery times and outcomes.

Patients typically recover from disc replacement surgery more quickly than fusion. ADR recovery is often measured in weeks rather than months, with many patients able to stand and walk within 24 hours of the surgery. In fact, at our hospital, we usually have our patients up and moving around (in a very safe and supported fashion) within 18 hours of surgery. On the other hand, traditional lumbar fusion can require protracted recovery times in order to allow proper solidification at the fusion site. Remember, although the surgery is called "fusion," the surgery does not immediately fuse the spine. Instead, the surgical procedure puts appropriate hardware and grafting material in place to *allow* fusion. Rods, cages, screws and plates serve to hold the vertebrae in a fixed position long enough for the two vertebrae to grow toward each other. Initial fusion takes place over a period of a few months, but the fusion is still relatively soft. It will actually solidify more over the next 12-18 months. This is one of the reasons fusion patients can have protracted (and sometimes painful) recovery times. Naturally, actual recovery time will depend on the individual patient, the procedure performed, the surgical team and many more factors.

Contrast this with people who have undergone disc replacement with our team. ADR recipients, even ones with ADR at multiple levels, are usually walking without assistance within one to two days and walking several *miles* a day within a week.

Some of them are even able to do miles of *bike riding* in the 7-10 days following surgery. And whereas fusion surgery takes months and sometimes a year or more to create a solid fusion, the M6 device we use creates a firm joint with the vertebrae almost immediately and ultimately fuses with the vertebrae in only six weeks. When we look at long-term recovery, our ADR patients complete most of their recovery in the first 100 days.

Following artificial disc replacement, most patients can lead a completely normal life. Patients can even return to strenuous exercise and sports in most circumstances, something that is often precluded following spinal fusion. We are continuously reminded by our patients about the excellent results possible with ADR. We have patients who have returned to all sorts of activities, including:

- Snow skiing
- Water Polo
- Body surfing
- Sledding
- Water skiing
- Horseback riding
- ATV and motorcycle riding
- Cycling
- Long-distance running
- Open water swimming
- Basketball
- Volleyball
- Mountain biking
- Tennis
- Golf
- Climbing
- Triathlon
- And more!

This isn't to say that every patient who receives disc replacement is going to perform such activities. There are many factors involved. But we frequently hear back from our patients who tell us of the wonderful things they can do.

We have had patients who have gone on to do professional cycling and even Ironman Triathlons following multi-level disc replacement. In case you aren't familiar with the Ironman

Triathlon, it consists of a 2.4-mile swim followed by 112-mile bicycle ride and a marathon 26.2-mile run, without a break. This is commonly called "one of the most difficult one-day sporting events in the world." (Ironman Triathlon, 2016)

While these examples are exciting to consider, and we are proud of them, there is a far more important measure for many people: a return to work. The vast majority of artificial disc recipients, at least in our experience, are able to return to work, some within only a week or two following surgery. Nothing gives me greater joy than to see someone who was productive and healthy before an injury then return to health and productivity. This helps not just the patients but their families too. Fathers and mothers are now better able to support and care for their children, spouses, and extended family. This is critical and probably the most important thing about what we do.

Though recoveries and outcomes vary from person to person and can be influenced by a great number of factors, we are continually encouraged by the successes our patients share with us.

LUMBAR AND CERVICAL DISC REPLACEMENT

Initially, disc replacement was only performed in the lumbar spine. Development of successful solutions for the cervical spine took longer. The natural discs in the cervical spine are much smaller than in the lumbar spine, and it was more difficult to create effective hardware. Fortunately, several artificial disc options now exist for the cervical spine.

Surgical indications for the cervical spine are similar to those for the lumbar spine and include degenerative disc disease or discogenic disease. We most often see these problems at the levels of C5-6 and C6-7, but consideration for disc replacement can be given for much of the cervical spine. Symptoms that point to a need for disc replacement include not just neck pain but also pain, numbness or tingling that extends into one or more upper extremities. Some ADR patients come to us with severe symptoms in the arms. Others come with numbness extending into the jaw or face. All of these symptoms may point to a need for intervention.

Cervical disc replacement, like lumbar ADR, is performed with an anterior, or frontal, approach. Approaching the cervical spine from the front shares the same advantages as in the lumbar spine. The existing, damaged disc can be easily seen and therefore removed. The artificial disc can be put in place from the side opposite the spinal canal. This means the surgeon can insert the new disc without having an impact on the spinal cord. The anterior approach allows the surgeon access to nearly all of the cervical spine.

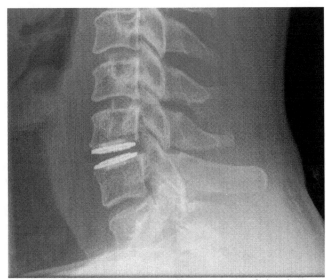

Cervical ADR (the non-metallic portions of the device are not visible on the xray)

The incision itself is very small, often less than four or five centimeters (under two inches). When sutured with a plastic surgery stitch, the surgical site heals with little to no scarring. In fact, should you need such a surgery, you can minimize and nearly eliminate any scar simply by following the surgeon's instructions post-operatively.

At present, my surgical team has completed more than 1,000 cervical disc replacement surgeries. Whereas cervical disc replacement used to be a rare or infrequent event, we now perform these procedures as much as several times a week.

Interestingly, although cervical solutions were late in coming, recovery from cervical disc replacement is easier than lumbar. Patients are not only up and walking around the day after surgery; they are also exhibiting near-normal range of motion of the neck. In fact, many patients are very pleasantly surprised at the lack of symptoms following surgery.

LUMBAR AND CERVICAL ADR IN THE SAME SURGERY

Many people are surprised to learn that lumbar and cervical disc replacement can be performed on the same day. Their surprise is understandable. Many traditional spinal surgeries are very invasive procedures that require many hours to perform. To perform such a lengthy surgery on the lumbar spine and then turn around and do it again on the cervical spine might seem excessive.

One of the great advantages to disc replacement, however, is that it can be performed quite quickly if it is done by an experienced surgical team. A typical one-to-two level fusion performed by a surgeon will often take two to three hours. A one-to-two level disc replacement performed by our surgical team takes only 1.25 hours on average. Our team is so skilled at disc replacement that each member of the team knows his or her role backwards and forwards. We can approach each surgery with skill and precision because we have done these procedures *literally thousands of times.* Thus, surgeries are performed more accurately and more efficiently. The increased accuracy leads to better outcomes and lower complication rates. The increased time savings allows us to perform both lumbar and cervical disc replacement in the same surgery without keeping the patient under anesthesia for too long.

We can approach each surgery with skill and precision because we have done these procedures literally thousands of times.

Disc replacement is also a mini-invasive surgery, performed through a very limited opening and with very minimal blood loss. Our typical lumbar ADR patient loses less than 200 milliliters of blood. That is less than seven ounces. To put this in perspective, that is 25% less than the blood loss in the typical oral surgery according to one study (Moenning, Bussard, Lapp, & Garrison, 1995). Such little blood loss means there is little-to-no additional stress put on the body if a second, cervical procedure is performed at the same time. And cervical ADR involves even less blood loss, only about 50 ml.

Our surgical team also employs the "Cell Saver" device. Most of the blood lost during surgery is collected in a centrifuge. If for some reason there is more than normal blood loss, we have the option of spinning and cleaning the patient's blood and giving it back to him or her. This reduces the impact of surgery and helps avoid any need for additional blood transfusion with someone else's blood.

Lastly, recovery from disc replacement is much easier than from other spine surgeries. Most people would agree that it would be extremely difficult to recover from lumbar fusion and cervical fusion at the same time. Traditionally speaking, surgeons would demand that a patient fully recover from the first fusion before even considering a second fusion procedure. But this is not the case with disc replacement when performed by an experienced team. The recovery process following disc replacement is so much easier than with fusion that getting cervical and lumbar disc replacement at the same time poses no dramatic problems.

The brief duration of surgery, minimal blood loss, and ease of recovery make simultaneous lumbar and cervical disc replacement not only feasible but often desirable. Patients who have degenerative disc disease in both their lower back and neck can often benefit from having both procedures done on the same day. We have performed these dual surgeries many times. It is not at all uncommon now for a patient to have one or two discs replaced in the lumbar spine and have another disc (or more) replaced in the cervical spine. In one instance, an emergency room physician required disc replacement at multiple levels. He felt so comfortable with our team and procedures that he had us replace three lumbar discs and four cervical discs on the same day. He had excellent results. While this is not typical, it demonstrates that combined lumbar and cervical surgeries are safe and reasonable where indicated.

He felt so comfortable with our team and procedures that he had us replace three lumbar discs and four cervical discs on the same day.

DIAGNOSES COMMONLY TREATED WITH DISC REPLACEMENT

Disc replacement can be used to treat a variety of diagnoses, and I have listed some of them below. When it comes to diagnoses, keep in mind that some disorders will have more than one name. For instance, what we call herniated nucleus pulposus is also commonly called a herniated disc or HNP. If you are having back problems, see if your diagnosis is on this list:

- Degenerative Disc Disease with or without herniated nucleus pulposus, with or without neuroforaminal stenosis, and without/with pseudo- or radicular syndrome
- Herniated or bulging disc
- Postnucleo-/Post-discotomy/Post-Discectomy Syndrome with progressing Degenerative Disc Disease
- Spinal canal stenosis caused by soft tissue (bulging), cervical possibly also with myelopathy
- Adjacent Level Disease/Adjacent Level Syndrome
- Slight segmental misalignment
- Initial degenerative spondylolisthesis without stenosis

Other factors need to be considered. These may include age, other illnesses that may be present, neurological problems, and more. For this reason, you should always seek a personalized evaluation by a surgeon who is very experienced in disc replacement.

THE EVOLUTION OF DISC REPLACEMENT

Early efforts with disc replacement included implantation of a ball in place of the original disc. A Swedish doctor, Dr. Fernström, pioneered this technique in Europe in the 1960's. The results were not well received in the surgical community. While other surgeons made additional efforts with metallic spheres throughout the 60's and 70's, there was limited success. Most devices were discontinued after only 10-15 surgeries.

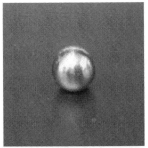

Fernström Ball, the first artificial "disc"

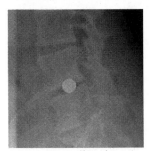

Fernström Ball in the spine

The breakthrough in disc replacement came in the 1980's at Charite University Hospital in Berlin, where I studied and operated for many years. Karin Büttner-Janz and Kurt Schellnack, under the supervision of Hartmut Zippel, developed a device now referred to as the SB Charite and took this through several generations. The first two generations of the device worked well, but real success was had in the 3rd generation. The SB Charite disc was the first disc to be implanted over 1000 times. This device did not receive approval from the U.S. Food and Drug Administration (FDA) for use in the U.S. until 2004 and then only for single-level surgeries at the L4-S1 level (FDA, 2004 Device Approvals, 2004). Interestingly, by then, the device was considered obsolete by many surgeons in Europe, who had moved on to use more advanced hardware. Over a 20-year period, more than 30,000 SB Charite devices were implanted worldwide.

Cervical devices were more difficult to develop than lumbar devices due to the smaller size. The first successful cervical device to be widely used was the Prestige. Although developed and used as far back as 2003 and 2004, it did not receive approval by the FDA until 2007 (FDA, 2007).

In the meantime, other devices were developed, including the ProDisc (lumbar and cervical), Maverick (lumbar), Active-L (lumbar), and Mobi-C (cervical). As of the writing of this book, the ProDisc and Activ-L have received U.S. FDA approval, but only for single-level use. The Mobi-C, and more recently the Prestige LP, have been approved for two-level use under limited conditions (FDA, 2007 Device Approvals, 2007). The Charite is no longer supported by its manufacturer. The Maverick was apparently barred from the U.S. market (at least initially) over patent infringement issues. Other devices continued to be developed.

In 2005, our team started working with the M6 device from U.S.-based Spinal Kinetics. I had the honor of being the surgeon to perform the very first implant of the cervical version of the M6 device in Europe. In fact, at that time, only 15 devices had been implanted worldwide (Spinal Kinetics, 2009). I was very excited about the M6 because it was the first disc to truly mimic the natural disc, providing both motion and shock absorption. I also had the honor of assisting Spinal Kinetics in developing the surgical tools and procedures for the M6. Since that time, I have installed thousands of the devices and have completed the first clinical studies charting two-year results within a large population of patients. I have also had the honor of training surgeons from around the world in the implantation of the M6.

Oddly enough, though disc replacement has had a substantial history in Europe, it is still relatively new in the U.S. and Canada. And though a few devices have been approved for limited use by the FDA, some U.S.-based insurance companies still consider it experimental. This is very unfortunate given the long-term results European surgeons have been seeing for decades now.

TYPES OF ARTIFICIAL DISC IMPLANTS

As of the writing of this book, there are several different artificial discs on the market. They fall into three major categories: *Unconstrained, semi-constrained,* and *fully constrained* (or simply "constrained").

Unconstrained devices have two or more parts that move freely in relation to each other. One example of this is the SB Charite III disc. This consists of metal endplates attached to the vertebrae above and below the removed disc. An extremely dense polyethylene core is then inserted between these plates. The design allows the parts to move freely in relation to each other in order to restore motion to the spine. Hence, this type of device is considered "unconstrained."

The Charite device received FDA approval in 2004 but only for use in patients with single-level degenerative disc disease in the area of L4-S1 (FDA, 2004 Device Approvals, 2004). As I discuss elsewhere in this book, our experience is that the majority of patients have multi-level disc disease and require replacement of two or more discs, so this FDA limitation is troubling for many patients.

Furthermore, the challenge with most unconstrained devices is they allow too much movement, sometimes much more than a normal human disc. The additional movement can place stresses on the facets of the vertebrae surrounding the implant. These bony portions of the vertebrae limit motion in a normal spine. Much of the motion-limiting function in a healthy spine is performed by the sinews and fibers in a healthy disc. In the case of unconstrained devices, there is no limiting function except the bony facets. As a result, these facets undergo unusual stress levels, and degeneration and wear of these facets may be accelerated.

Another non-constrained device now available in Europe is the Triadyme from Dymicron. This consists of industrial diamond dust that is molded and pressed into two complementary structures. The parts are harder than any metal. Interestingly, though the two parts move freely over each other and are therefore technically "unconstrained," the engineered design actually limits motion to attempt to imitate the limited motion in a natural disc. It is a very well-engineered device. As of the writing of this book, it is also a very new device, and I will be monitoring the results as it is tested and used more widely.

Semi-Constrained devices include several components, at least two of which are physically attached to each other. As such, these attached pieces cannot move out of position in relation to each other. An example of a semi-constrained disc replacement is the ProDisc. This device is a "ball and socket" device, much like an artificial hip is a ball and socket. One piece containing a metal endplate and plastic ball is attached to one vertebra, and the other piece containing a metal concave end plate socket is attached to the other vertebra. The two halves are not physically attached to each other but rely instead on the pressure of the spine and surrounding tissues to keep the two parts in contact. The ProDisc has been used for more than ten years. This device was not approved by the FDA for use in the U.S. until 2006, and then only for single-level use (FDA, 2006).

Like unconstrained devices, the semi-constrained devices often allow too much movement. They are, therefore, sometimes associated with accelerated wear on the facet joints of the surrounding vertebrae.

One challenge for most artificial disc devices is that few mimic the shock-absorbing ability of a natural disc. This is true of the ProDisc. The two mating surfaces lack any substantial cushion. For this reason, and because of the complications from hypermobility, many surgeons in countries where disc replacement is performed have moved on to other devices. However, because of the limitations of the FDA, the ProDisc remains one of the few lumbar devices available in the U.S.

Fully constrained discs are those where all elements of the artificial disc are joined together. The M6 device from Spinal Kinetics is an example. The M6 device is composed of two titanium parts joined together by a flexible, fiber core. All three portions remain attached to each other and therefore cannot come apart. This connectivity decreases the likelihood of complications due to separation of the parts, and it also limits the motion of the artificial disc. At the same time, the M6 device mimics the natural disc in that it allows limited "translation" movement. Translation describes the natural motion of the vertebrae sliding slightly forward, backward, or sideways over the natural disc. This limited motion aids in the flexibility of the spine without negatively impacting strength. This same limited "translation" motion is a key feature of the M6 device. The M6, in fact, is called M6 because it allows all six of the qualities of motion present in a natural human disc.

6 Motions of a Disc

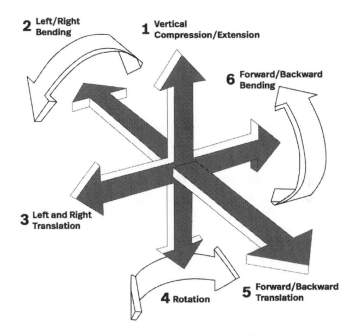

THE SIX QUALITIES OF MOTION:

1. Shock absorption (Compression and decompression of the spine)
2. Bending to one side or the other (lateral flexion)
3. Left and right "translation"
4. Rotation (twisting of the spine to left or right)
5. Forward and backward "translation"
6. Bending forward and backward (flexion and extension)

At this time, we have installed thousands of the M6 devices. In fact, as of this writing, we have installed over 5,000 implants in the lumbar and cervical spine. We have had excellent results with extremely low complication rates across the board. In the very few instances when complications have arisen, they have not been due to any failure of the device but instead to the normal complications that can arise with any surgical procedure. Revision has been needed in less than 1% of our cases. See my chapter about short-and long-term studies of disc replacement for more information.

The M6 is, unfortunately, unavailable for use in the U.S. and Canada at this time. The M6-C (the cervical version of the M6) is undergoing trials for FDA approval at present. However, when it ultimately gets approved in the U.S., the FDA will still limit its use to single-level cervical procedures. Our research shows that the average patient requires intervention at more than one level. Statistically, lumbar patients average 1.6 implants, and cervical patients average 1.75 implants. Given this information, the fact that FDA approval will almost certainly be limited to single-level use is very unfortunate. For a more detailed discussion, see my chapter entitled "Where Can I Get ADR or Hybrid Intervention?"

IS DISC REPLACEMENT ALWAYS THE RIGHT SOLUTION?

Artificial disc replacement is an excellent option for the treatment of many spinal conditions, but it is not appropriate in all cases. First, ADR should only be considered if appropriate conservative measures have been employed. We never want to rush into surgery if non-surgical steps can be an effective measure. Medication, exercise, physical therapy, and other treatment methods all have their place and should be employed before surgery is explored.

Second, there are times where surgery is indicated but ADR is not. When properly installed, the top and bottom parts of the artificial disc will ultimately fuse to the surrounding vertebrae. But if the surrounding vertebrae are themselves damaged or weak, then ADR may not be appropriate. It does not help to implant a very strong and durable artificial disc if it cannot effectively fuse to the vertebrae. The device may move around or slip out of place. For this reason, people with low bone density can be poor candidates for ADR. Those who have damaged vertebrae above or below the site of the desired artificial disc may also be precluded. Deformities of the spine and what we call "macro-instabilities" can also preclude disc replacement.

Unfortunately, prior spine surgery *can* also be a barrier to disc replacement, but this depends greatly on the type of surgery performed. While ADR can often be performed with those who have undergone micro-discectomy or discotomy, surgeries that have altered the surrounding vertebra can be problematic. It ultimately comes down to whether the disc implant can safely and permanently adhere to the surrounding vertebrae and if the vertebrae are solid and stable enough for the implant to function properly.

The benefits of disc replacement are too high, and the potential complications of these other surgeries too serious, for you to make this decision without exploring all your options.

Another factor often considered is the current disc height of the location to be treated. Normal disc height is the distance between vertebrae when separated by a healthy, non-compressed disc. While some medical professionals believe that disc replacement is only appropriate when the disc height is at least 50% of normal, our extensive experience shows this plays only a minor role. The loss of disc height is not as important as any damage or deformity (arthrosis, stenosis, etc) that may have occurred in the joint. The decisive factor is whether or not the joint can be re-mobilized (or re-spaced) in surgery. If this is the case, then normal disc height can be restored and an implant can be put in place, even if the pre-operative disc height was less than 50% of normal.

A prior and stable fusion at the proposed surgery level will eliminate the possibility of an artificial disc being put in place. However, if the fusion was performed in the last six months and the fusion has not yet solidified, it may be possible for a disc replacement to be done instead. In such cases, the fusion hardware is usually removed and an artificial disc is implanted. This occurs in only exceptional cases.

Whether disc replacement is appropriate for you is a very important decision and one that should be made in consultation with a qualified surgeon, preferably one that is very experienced in disc replacement. If you are considering fusion or a more temporary solution like discectomy or discotomy, you owe it to yourself to speak with a surgeon about disc replacement. The benefits of disc replacement are too high, and the potential complications of these other surgeries too serious, for you to make this decision without exploring all your options.

If you would like a second opinion from me and my highly experienced surgical team, simply email your full name and email address to evaluation@enande.com. We will commence the steps for an in-depth, comprehensive evaluation right away.

DISC REPLACEMENT RESEARCH

Artificial Disc Replacement procedures have been subjected to rigorous study and analysis. Because of my role in early disc replacement surgeries, and because of our ongoing surgical practice, we have had the privilege of being part of many of these studies.

We recently presented the results of a two-year study on the use of the M6 artificial disc, the goal of which was to study and present how patients fare two years after single-level and multi-level disc replacement. The study is called *Two Year, Multi-Center Outcomes for the Treatment of Degenerative Disc Disease in the Lumbar Spine Using a Novel, Compressible Core Prosthesis* and was conducted by our team of surgeons at two different surgical hospitals. The results were impressive. Here are some of them:

We studied 83 patients for two years following surgery to gauge pre- and post-surgical pain using an industry-standard measure called the Oswestry Disability Index (ODI).   The ODI system allows patients to describe their intensity of pain, ability to lift, ability to care for oneself, ability to walk, ability to sit, sexual function, ability to stand, social life, sleep quality, and ability to travel. The scores for all questions are calculated to obtain the index, ranging from 0 to 100 (Oswestry Disability Index, 2016).   The ODI is widely regarded as the ideal tool for measuring lumbar spine pain and disability (National Council for Osteopathic Research, 2012).

Patients are scored in the following ranges:

0-20	Minimal disability
21-40	Moderate disability
41-60	Severe disability
61-80	Crippling back pain
81-100	Bed-bound or exaggerating symptoms

Using this index as an objective measure, we discovered that both single- and multi-level ADR recipients experienced very significant relief and had better function after surgery. You can see the results on this table:

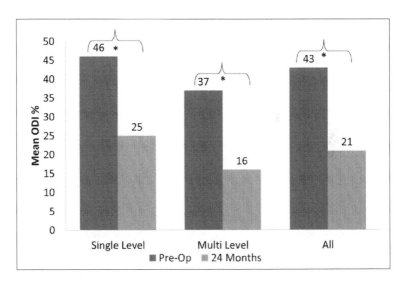

As part of this study, patients rated themselves prior to surgery using the self-questionnaire in the Oswestry Disability Index (ODI). Their scores were calculated, which placed them in one of the five disability categories: minimal, moderate, severe, crippled, or bed bound. Two years after surgery, this was repeated. Prior to surgery, 34% of our sample group were moderately disabled, and 45% were severely disabled. Another 13% were crippled, and 2% were bed bound. Only 6% had "minimal" disability prior to surgery. Two years after the surgery, this had all changed! The percentage of people who were moderately disabled, severely disabled and crippled dropped significantly, just as we hoped. The majority of patients moved from moderate or severely disabled (or worse) to minimal. The percentage of bed bound patients dropped by 100%. Though we had some bed-bound patients prior to surgery, we had *zero* bed-bound patients after two years.

The following table shows the dramatic improvements patients had following single level ADR surgery:

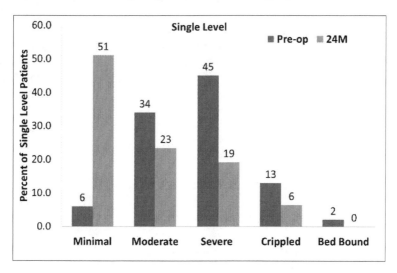

As for those with multi-level disc replacement surgery, we had even *better* results. This may be surprising to some people. When patients are told they need multi-level fusion, there is great fear and trepidation. This is understandable given the potential complications and long-term problems that can occur with traditional fusion. And the more levels that need to be fused often signal a more severe condition and, perhaps, more opportunities for short and long-term problems following fusion.

The vast majority of patients moved from moderately or severely disabled to the category of minimal.

Our studies, however, show something different when it comes to artificial disc replacement. Prior to surgery, 48% of our multi-level study group of patients were described as moderately disabled, and 30% were severely disabled; 3% were crippled, and another 3% were bed bound. Twenty-four months after surgery, the results were impressive. The vast majority of patients moved from moderately or severely disabled to the category of minimal. And though we started with six patients that were crippled or bed-bound, *none* of the patients were crippled or bed bound two years after disc replacement.

Here are the results in table format.

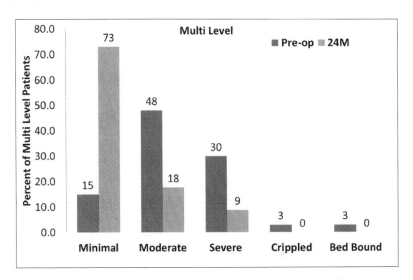

The results of the study, the first of its kind for the M6 device, show that the M6 is a highly effective tool for treating degenerative disc disease. Patients experienced significantly reduced pain levels and far lower levels of disability.

Of course, this study just confirms what we have been seeing in our clinic for years since commencing use of this device in 2005. We have seen firsthand how patients come into the hospital with severe disabilities and leave with a new lease on life. Although I won't call this typical, we have had patients walking six or seven hours a day only five days after surgery. It is not unheard of for our patients to be riding bikes a week or two post-op. Of course, everyone's result is different, but we have seen incredible results from both single-level and multi-level ADR. And now we have this two-year study to quantify and qualify our results.

But what about the long-term results? What about *after* two years? Although this study was the first to study the two-year results with the M6 device, the patients are being monitored for a five-year study as well. We can already see a positive trend line, as patients continue to improve.

TEN YEARS WITH THE M6 ARTIFICIAL DISC

We started working with the M6 device in 2005. We helped Spinal Kinetics, the manufacturer, to develop the tools and procedures necessary to implant this device into the spine. Today, Spinal Kinetics reports more than 43,000 M6 discs have been implanted in 27 countries across six continents. These surgeons are using the tools and procedures we developed. In fact, many of these surgeons have received training and instruction from our team of doctors.

These surgeons are using the tools and procedures we developed.

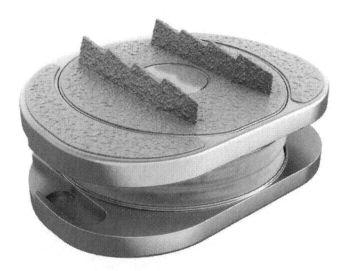

The M6 from Spinal Kinetics

As of the writing of this book, we now have more than a decade of experience with this excellent device. We have the joy of hearing from our patients on a regular basis. They call us and send us letters and emails. They send us pictures of themselves performing tasks they just couldn't tolerate before surgery. They pay us the very highest compliment by referring their friends and family members for surgery. In fact, as of the writing of this book, most our clients come through personal referrals.

We have seen firsthand how disc replacement has restored not just spines but *lives.* Here are just a few examples:

Curtis Smith from Fresno, California underwent a 3-level lumbar disc replacement in May of 2014. Prior to surgery, he was *living on the floor* of his home, unable to sit or stand long enough to either work or do the things people normally do around the house. His pain was so bad that he slept on the floor and even took his meals on the floor. Several doctors told him he needed a 4-level fusion. At age 41, Curtis was worried about the long-term results he would have with most of his lumbar spine fused. On the recommendation of one of our patients, Curtis reached out to our clinic and researched his options.

A few months after surgery, Curtis' life had changed. He wasn't living on the floor anymore. He had returned to work without any limitations, and he was living a very active lifestyle. A year after surgery, he could zip line, play basketball, water ski, and play in the ocean with his kids, all things he had been unable to do just one year prior. 18 months after surgery, he returned to snow skiing as well. Curtis has his life back.

Jeff Gute is a farmer and auto enthusiast from the Central U.S. Prior to cervical disc replacement with the M6, he spent more than two years unable to turn his neck to one side or the other. He also had excruciating pain. The day after surgery, Jeff could turn and twist his neck freely. Three days after surgery, he was spotted on the lawn outside the hospital, kicking a ball around with another patient's son. A month after surgery, Jeff was feeding his cows and driving his tractor.

Jeff sent us this note less than two months after surgery:

> *My recovery has been smooth and easy.... The amount of relief and comfort I now feel is liberating. I haven't been able to turn my head for a couple of years without pain and restrictions. Now I feel brand new!! I'm able to get back to my hobbies such as farming and working on my hotrod and my Harley chopper. I'm getting my MOJO back.   Jeff*

We have lots of stories like these. But don't read these and other case studies and think that recovery is a "walk in the park" all the time (although walking in the park is literally part of the recovery process!). Recovery from major surgery takes time. Progress is often slow. And every patient recovers at different rates. While some patients want to get up and start walking only hours after surgery, others take a day or two to get moving around. Some patients return to work within weeks of surgery, and others take longer. All patients experience some level of pain and stiffness following surgery. Symptoms typically subside over time. This is all normal and to be expected following spine surgery.

HYBRID INTERVENTION

In cases where disc replacement is not appropriate, spinal fusion may indeed be the best option. Wonderful advances have been made in the world of spinal fusion, with improved techniques and better hardware. When performed by a highly-skilled surgeon and experienced surgical team, fusion can be quite effective. But even in these circumstances, disc replacement may play a very important role. There are times where a surgeon may recommend a multiple-level fusion where the best option may actually be a combination of fusion and artificial disc replacement, what we call hybrid intervention.

One of the greatest challenges with traditional fusion is that the fusion hardware causes a previously mobile and flexible portion of the spine to become completely rigid. While this helps to stop the pain and nerve impingement originating at the fused level, it places substantial, additional strain on the discs above and below the fusion site. These discs take additional stress because these joints are essentially called upon to make up for the inflexibility of the fused portion of the spine. Over time, the discs near the fused levels begin to deteriorate and compress. Soon, the person with a traditional fusion finds him or herself requiring additional fusion at these adjacent levels. This has become so common that we now have a new disease called Adjacent Segment Syndrome or Adjacent Segment Disease. Sadly, even when the fusion is performed by an excellent surgical team, more than 15% of patients require additional surgical intervention at adjacent levels within only 10 years.

A better solution is often a hybrid intervention, where we combine fusion with artificial disc replacement.   In such circumstances, our surgical team works together to fuse the spine at one or more levels while implanting artificial discs at one or more adjacent levels.   While this is a more complex surgery and results in longer recovery periods than disc replacement alone, this is usually far superior to a multi-level fusion in many ways. The patient is left with much more motion and flexibility in the spine.   In addition, the added stress and strain that a fusion normally transmits to the discs above and below a fusion site are now borne in many cases by the artificial disc. The implant is often better able to withstand the added "wear and tear" than a natural disc can.   For instance, the combination of rigid and flexible materials in the M6 artificial disc has been tested to more than 30 million cycles.   Such an implant will likely outlast the patient and can certainly endure any additional stresses far better than the natural disc, thereby staving off Adjacent Segment Disease. Therefore, patients that have undergone these hybrid surgeries usually have a far better result in the short term *and* in the long term than if they underwent multiple-level fusion without disc replacement.

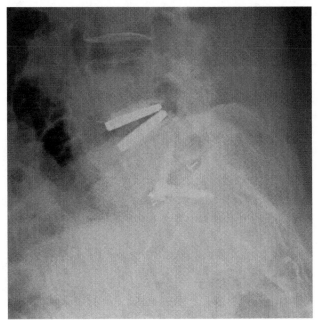

X-ray of hybrid intervention (lumbar ADR and anterior fusion)

Unfortunately, dual solutions such as these are often unavailable in the U.S and Canada. Very few surgeons have substantial experience combining these two different procedures. Because of the FDA's limitation to only one-to two-level ADR (depending on the device indications), a person who needs three levels addressed must have one or more levels fused when perhaps disc replacement would have been appropriate at one or more of these levels.

Although many patients might prefer *only* disc replacement over a combination of disc replacement and fusion, hybrid intervention is sometimes the best possible solution. As we discussed in the section on disc replacement, there are times where disc replacement is not an appropriate choice. If there is too much instability of the surrounding vertebrae or poor bone density, installation of an artificial disc is not the right choice. In these cases, fusion at that level may be needed. But the insertion of an artificial disc implant at adjoining levels is usually far superior to additional levels of fusion. A person requiring treatment at three levels can now have a fusion at one level and disc replacement at the others. This allows near-normal motion of the spine since only one level is fused. This may also mean faster recovery and less likelihood of long-term complications.

If multiple-level fusion has been recommended for you or a loved one by a surgeon who is not highly experienced with both fusions and disc replacements, proceed cautiously and get the answers you need.

There are clear, scientific indications that determine when disc replacement is appropriate and when it is not. A surgeon who has performed thousands of disc replacements and thousands of fusions is well equipped to make this determination in an objective manner.

If multiple-level fusion has been recommended for you or a loved one by a surgeon who is *not* highly experienced with both fusions *and disc replacements*, proceed cautiously and get the answers you need. Never be afraid to get a second (or third) opinion, perhaps from a surgeon who is not confined by the artificial limitations of the FDA. Consider all your options, and explore disc replacement along with hybrid intervention. Your best outcome will rely on the proper surgery performed by the proper surgeon with the proper surgical team.

COMPLIMENTARY EVALUATION

You may already know you want to explore disc replacement or hybrid intervention. Or you may know you want a second opinion from me and my highly experienced surgical team. If so, I want to extend to you, free of charge, the opportunity for an in-depth, comprehensive evaluation. Simply email your full name and email address to evaluation@enande.com, and we will respond right away.

WHEN FUSION IS REQUIRED

Although treatment with artificial disc replacement is usually far superior to fusion when ADR is appropriate, fusion is sometimes the best option. Spinal fusion has developed negative connotations and a poor reputation because fusion has been associated with decreased mobility and higher complication rates when compared to ADR and other less-invasive surgery. In reality, modern fusion techniques can be a very effective remedy. Procedures such as isolated anterior fusions (ALIF), anterior-posterior fusions (360° fusion), posterior fusion with or without cages (PLIF, TLIF etc.), as well as the complex corrective fusions can effectively transform a painful disease of the spine into a painless or pain-free situation in which load-bearing is possible and quality of life is improved. The development of minimally invasive approach techniques and the development of implants in the last 30 years show an increasing reduction in complication rates with a significant improvement of clinical success.

Results, however, are highly dependent on the experience of the surgeon. There are some surgeons in the medical community who perform such surgeries on an infrequent basis. Most spinal surgeons perform less than 100 surgeries a year. On the other hand, there are a few "centers of excellence" around the world where highly specialized teams of surgeons perform hundreds of these surgeries a year. Because they perform surgery so often, they have perfected the entire process. This process involves the highest of quality and the best possible practices at every step, from evaluation and diagnosis, through surgery, and all the way to recovery and follow-up care. It involves skilled and experienced team members not only in the surgical suite but also in the recovery room and in the hospital as a whole, along with state-of-the art techniques for infection control, physiotherapy, and more. Because of this effective team environment, patients of these centers of excellence have some of the lowest complication rates in the world, the fastest recovery times, and the best long-term results.

If you have been told that you require cervical or lumbar fusion, you should seek out one of these centers of excellence for a second opinion. The odds are very high that you may find you are a candidate for artificial disc replacement or hybrid intervention instead of traditional fusion. This would allow you to benefit from superior long-term results and a likelihood of returning to a normal life after surgery. Even if fusion is required at one or more levels, you may find that ADR can be employed to decrease the number of fused levels, providing you with the best possible outcome both in the short term and the long term. And should you learn that a traditional fusion truly is necessary, you will have the option of having it performed by a precision team including some of the best spinal surgeons in the world. Our team has extensive experience with both fusion and hybrid intervention. In fact, we have performed over 5,000 fusions (lumbar and cervical), and we have performed over 600 hybrid interventions. *Very* few teams can make such a claim. If you would like our team of surgeons to take a look at your case, just email your name and phone number to evaluation@enande.com. A member of our team will get back to you.

You owe it to yourself to get the best possible outcome from your surgery, and that starts with a second opinion from the right surgical team.

Nobody should undergo *any* surgery without a second opinion. When it comes to your spine, the central structure of your body, this is doubly true. The decision to undergo spinal surgery, and which type of surgery, is one of the most important decisions you will ever have to make in your life. Perhaps equally important is which surgeon will do your surgery. You want to make sure you get as much information as possible to help you make these decisions. You owe it to yourself to get the best possible outcome from your surgery, and that starts with a second opinion from the right surgical team.

CASE STUDY: JOHN DEVERE

Two-level lumbar artificial disc recipient, with surgery performed in 2005:

I am a physical education teacher, and I also coach water polo and swimming. I've been athletic all my life. When I was younger, I got very active in rodeo, swam and played water polo. I was a High School "All-American" in water polo. After high school, I got into riding bikes and then became a professional triathlete.

I blew my back out in 2002. I had just qualified to represent the USA at the World Triathlon Championships in Mexico. But I fell while playing ultimate frisbee with my P.E. students. I knew something was wrong right away, like an electrical shock that went out my spine. I went home that day and didn't come back to work for about two weeks. One night, I went to go to the bathroom and ended up on the floor, and I stayed on the floor for about four hours till the ambulance came and got me. That is how it started.

I had to back out of the World Championships because I was in agony. I was ultimately able to go back to work, but I was working with constant pain. It got to the point where I would sometimes break down and sob uncontrollably because of the pain. I use the word 'sob' over the word 'cry' because when you sob, it's an emotional weeping to where you just can't take this anymore. I can remember telling my wife, "Something's got to change. Give me my gun. I'll go in the other room. Something's got to change, and it's got to change now. I'm not doing this anymore."

Around this time, I discovered total disc replacement and Dr. Ritter-Lang. I had been on the web constantly, trying to find solutions for my incredible pain. I literally spent hundreds of hours looking at what was available. At that point, I found Dr. Ritter-Lang. In 2005, I underwent two-level disc replacement at L4-L5 and L5-S1.

CASE STUDY: JOHN DEVERE (CONT.)

The improvement was immediate.

Though I had pain associated with the surgery, my unbearable nerve pain was gone within days. In fact, I felt so good that I went back to my job as a P.E. teacher and swim coach only 3 or 4 days after returning to the U.S. I think I took a total of 3 weeks off for the surgery, including travel.

I think I was 47 at that time, and I went back to riding my bike. Within a year and a half, I was racing at the top professional levels again. It was incredible. Though I sometimes had some mild back pain, it was nothing like I had before. And I was not only able to work but also race professionally once more. In fact, I was riding about 300 miles a week on top of working 9 or 10 hours a day.

That ended in 2015, when I was 54. I was in a professional race when another racer ran into me in such a way that I went down really, really hard. I broke my shoulder in three places, broke the top of my femur off on my right side, and broke nine ribs. The ribs punctured my lung in seven different places, and on the way to the hospital, I actually coded because my lungs had filled up with blood so quickly. I was in ICU for a week after that accident and spent another three weeks in the hospital. I was in a wheelchair for six months after that.

But the one thing that really shocked me is that this horrible accident had no effect on my back and my artificial discs. They didn't move or break, and my back is wonderful. Recovering from all the other injuries has taken a long time, and I will feel the effects of the accident for the rest of my life. But I am incredibly grateful for the work performed by Dr. Ritter-Lang and his surgical team.

CASE STUDY: JOHN DEVERE (CONT.)

After more than a decade with artificial discs, I can say with confidence I made the correct choice. For this reason, I frequently refer people to Dr. Ritter-Lang and his team. In my opinion, they are the best in the world at what they do. And I am living proof of this.

John Devere, Clovis CA, USA

4

FREQUENTLY ASKED QUESTIONS ABOUT DISC REPLACEMENT

HOW LONG DOES DISC REPLACEMENT SURGERY TAKE?

THE LENGTH OF time it takes to complete Artificial Disc Replacement surgery can vary significantly depending on the skill and experience of the surgeon and the surgical team. The typical spinal surgeon who performs ADR a few times a month may take two or more hours for a single-level ADR procedure. On the other hand, if the surgery is being performed by a highly experienced surgeon and team, this time falls considerably. At our hospital, where we perform multiple ADR surgeries every week, a single-level ADR takes approximately one hour. A multi-level disc replacement is usually accomplished within 60 to 90 minutes. Even a hybrid procedure, where ADR and fusion are combined, takes our team only about 90-120 minutes, largely because of our experience and skill with these procedures.

This is very important if you or a loved one are considering spinal surgery. The amount of time you spend in surgery is critical to your recovery. The longer you are in surgery, the higher the chance for problems and complications. The shorter your surgery, the less blood loss you may sustain, the less time you are under anesthesia, and the lower your chance of infection. It stands to reason that the chance of infection increases the longer your surgery is underway. The sooner your wounds are closed and sutured, the better. You want to be exposed to potential complications for as little time as possible.

MRSA, or methicillin-resistant Staphylococcus aureus, is a very dangerous Hospital Acquired Infection. The U.S. Centers for Disease Controls tracks MRSA infection rates throughout the world. Although hospital acquired MRSA rates have fallen by 50% in the last decade, infection rates in the U.S. are still more than twice as high as Germany (CDDEP, 2016).

The short surgery times at our hospital are one of the reasons we have a very low infection rate. Our general infection rate is 1.8%, far below the average surgical suite. Hospital infection rates are carefully monitored in Germany, and tracking is mandated by law. The truth is, we have never had an instance of a primary infection following disc replacement surgery. While we have had the inevitable low-grade infections in a few cases, the occurrence has been less than 1 in 1,000.

While MRSA infection rates are quite high in the United States and Canada, we have essentially no MRSA cases at our hospital. This is for several reasons. First, MRSA occurence in Germany is far lower than in North America in general. Second, our surgical suite is in a specialty hospital that serves only orthopaedic patients. Because the hospital does not have an emergency room and does not take other types of patients, the risk of an MRSA infected patient being admitted are extremely low. Finally, we screen all patients for MRSA ahead of time. This helps protect all patients from contracting a MRSA infection.

WHERE CAN I GET ADR OR HYBRID INTERVENTION PERFORMED?

Unfortunately, your access to Artificial Disc Replacement and hybrid intervention may be hampered by your location. While ADR has been performed for decades in other parts of the world, the U.S. and Canada have been slow in coming up to speed with the procedures. This is not due to any specific problems with ADR or hybrid intervention but simply because of the regulatory processes and medical systems in these countries.

Currently, in the U.S., the most commonly used device is the ProDisc, which is approved for single-level use only. For a time, the ProDisc was one of the best artificial discs available. But it has not aged well, so to speak. In fact, by the time the ProDisc was approved for use in the U.S. by the Food and Drug Administration (FDA), it was already considered obsolete in Germany and other countries where disc replacement is frequently performed. Ongoing studies of the ProDisc show a higher than necessary complication rate along with concerns for facet arthrosis. Unlike the M6 device, which mimics the normal, limited motion of a natural disc, the ProDisc allows *more* than normal motion. This is one of those times when more is *not* better. The resulting hypermobility increases the stresses on the facets (portions of the vertebrae above and below the artificial disc). Over time, this can cause damage.

The ProDisc has also had a rough track record when it comes to the need for revision surgery. In fact, studies have shown that the device has required as much as 8.7% of the patients to have a second surgery within two to three years (Siepe, Mayer, Wiechert, & Korge, 2006). Yet the ProDisc is still used for single-level disc replacement in the U.S. and Canada.

Meanwhile, the M6 device, for instance, is used in 27 countries around the world, and over 43,000 devices have been implanted since it was released internationally in 2007. I had the honor of being the first surgeon ever to implant the M6-L (lumbar) artificial disc, and I have implanted thousands of them since. I was also the first surgeon in Europe to implant the M6-C (cervical) disc, two years before its general release. Fortunately, FDA testing is now underway for its use in the U.S. While it may be still several years before the device sees widespread use in the states, it seems highly likely that the M6 will become a valid treatment option for people there.

Sadly, there is an additional challenge. The FDA has been very slow to approve multi-level artificial disc replacement. A high percentage of patients require treatment at more than one level of the spine. A doctor's recommendation for a two or three-level fusion seems more and more common these days. For U.S. patients, though, only one lumbar level can be treated with ADR (typically in the form of a ProDisc). And, as of the writing of this book, only two cervical devices have been approved for multi-level use, and that only in limited circumstances (FDA, 2016).

The remaining level(s) must instead be fused, even when an additional level of disc replacement might be the best solution. While this is often better than *all* of the injured levels being fused, it does not compare well to the restored function and decreased pain that we see with multi-level disc replacement. There may come a time soon when multi-level ADR will be common in the U.S. and Canada, but, for now, surgeons in these countries are sadly limited in their treatment options.

Even though the M6 (which is actually made in the U.S.), is going through the FDA approval process, my sources indicate that, even when it is approved, it will still only be approved for *single-level* use. Frankly, common multi-level use of state-of-the-art artificial discs may be a decade or more away *in North America*. By the time the FDA has given approval for multi-level ADR with the M6, the *state of the art* may have advanced to other disc implants and techniques.

For these reasons, patients often travel outside North America for disc replacement. To get the best possible treatment, they engage in what some call "medical tourism." This term doesn't describe getting treatment while on vacation; instead it refers to a more and more common practice of traveling to the part of the world that holds the best solution.

Many people who own a car will seek out the "best" mechanic. How you personally determine which mechanic is "best" may vary, but many people will consider the mechanic's experience working on their model of car, the mechanic's state-of-the-art diagnostic equipment, and repair options. Price also may come into consideration. Well, the best mechanic for your car may not have his shop in your neighborhood. You might have to drive across town to seek repairs if you want "the best."

This is true for medical treatment too. The best medical solution may not be available in your neighborhood...or nation. By one estimate, 1.4 million people engaged in medical tourism in 2016 (Patients Beyond Borders, 2016). Whether they traveled for different treatment options, better care, or more affordable treatment, they all left their "neighborhood" and drove "across town" for medical care. In the case of spinal surgery options, the best surgeon, surgical team, hospital and devices may not be available where you live. Traveling abroad may be required.

Disc replacement has been performed for many years in Germany. While disc replacement may be available in other countries, it is my belief that spine treatment options in Germany are excellent. High levels of care, low infection rates, and state-of-the-art devices make Germany a very attractive alternative for disc replacement and spinal surgery in general.

WHAT ANESTHESIA IS REQUIRED FOR ADR?

Cervical disc replacement is usually performed under general anesthesia. While the agents may vary and can be administered in different ways, the outcome is to render the patient unconscious and ensure the patient experiences no pain during the procedure. An anthesiologist carefully monitors the patient to make sure the patient is comfortable and safe.

Lumbar disc replacement, however, allows another option: Epidural Anesthesia. Also called Peridural Anesthesia or PDA, this involves the injection of an anesthetic into the epidural portion of the spinal column. This can have the effect of eliminating all feeling from the level of the epidural down to the toes. Commonly used in childbirth, it is very useful for lumbar disc replacement as well.

Technically, a patient with an epidural could be completely awake during the surgery without any pain whatsoever. Generally, however, the patient is given a light general anesthesia to place them in a form of "twilight sleep." This is done mostly to relax the patient and put them only slightly under during the surgery.

This has several advantages. First, an application of a heavy general anesthetic causes a stress reaction in the body, with increased adrenaline and cortisone production. This can leave a patient tired for several days afterward as they recover from the anesthesia. An epidural with a weak general anesthetic, however, largely avoids this problem and allows the patient to be mobilized more quickly after surgery. This greatly speeds recovery.

Second, if needed, the surgeon can wake the patient during surgery to immediately check nerve function. This is not readily available with a strong general anesthetic.

Third, the epidural may help break a patient's ongoing chronic pain cycle in the lumbar spine. Many patients undergoing ADR have had pain for years, often without interruption. The epidural gives the pain receptors or pain memory a chance to reset, at least partially.

Fourth, an epidural allows the patient to minimalize the use of opioid pain medication going to the surgery and during recovery. This has many benefits, not the least of which is the decreased likelihood of addiction.

Finally, the epidural can be left in place after surgery for administration of pain medications directly to the spine. This helps with pain management and remobilization of patients. This also allows rapid weaning from any opioids.

HOW IMPORTANT IS SELECTION OF A SURGEON?

While many people are smart to take steps to choose the best surgeon, the decision-making should not stop there. The truth is that the correct surgical *team* and hospital are also extremely important. But let's start with the surgeon.

What should you look for in a surgeon?

Selecting the right surgeon for your procedure is perhaps the most important decision you can make, maybe even more important than the decision between disc replacement and fusion. Even the most wonderful hardware will not help you if it is not implanted properly. In fact, I would personally take old hardware or even fusion over the latest hardware installed by a surgeon who is inexperienced with that hardware.

But the best outcome does not start with the surgery. It starts with the proper diagnosis and then the proper method to address this diagnosis. This is critical. There are surgeons who are very adept at fusions but less adept at determining who really *needs* a fusion...and poor at other procedures that could be more beneficial. A great spinal surgeon is a great *evaluator* first. He or she should be able to take the time to consider all the many factors that go into a proper diagnosis. And this involves far more than reviewing x-rays or MRI studies. A detailed understanding of your symptoms, history, and other factors is equally (and sometimes *more*) important in making a proper diagnosis. *After all, a surgery, no matter how skillfully performed, is a failure if it is the wrong treatment.*

> A great spinal surgeon is a great evaluator first.

> A surgery, no matter how skillfully performed, is a failure if it is the wrong treatment.

If surgery is indeed the proper course of action, then you want a surgeon who is *extremely* adept and experienced with your surgical procedure, and a surgeon that performs this surgery on a very frequent basis. Sadly, 90% of spine surgeons perform less than 100 surgeries a year. By contrast, our surgical team of three lead surgeons average about 850 surgeries a year.

You also want to consider other factors regarding your surgeon. Does your surgeon explain the pros and cons of the recommended procedure? Does he or she discuss other alternatives? Does your surgeon explain the underlying pathology or cause of your condition and why this particular surgery is needed to correct it?

Does your surgeon train other physicians in disc replacement? If possible, does he or she participate in internationally recognized studies? Does he or she speak at surgical conferences or teach at university hospitals? All of these factors go into selecting the proper surgeon. Now onto the surgical team.

WHAT SHOULD I LOOK FOR IN A SURGICAL TEAM?

Next in importance is the surgical team. You want a surgical team that performs your surgery very often. Such a team is like a well-oiled machine. An efficient surgical team means less time under anesthesia, less blood loss, fewer complications, more rapid recovery, and *more complete* recovery following surgery. I cannot stress this too much. Discover how many disc replacements they have performed, and learn how many years they have been doing disc replacements.

Our team has performed so many disc replacements that the surgical nurses seem to read my mind. They know what to expect. I rarely even have to ask for a tool. The nurse has usually already picked up the tool, prepared it for me, and is standing there with it when I need it. This saves a tremendous amount of time. The other surgeons on the team know exactly what to do at the proper time. As you can imagine, spinal surgery can be a complex undertaking. Having additional, experienced hands is invaluable. And should any complications occur, the experienced team of nurses and surgeons knows just how to react, with efficiency and precision.

An efficient surgical team means less time under anesthesia, less blood loss, fewer complications, more rapid recovery, and more complete recovery following surgery.

There are those who have described the activity in the surgical suite like an orchestra, with all the instruments playing their own notes and tones but in a way that comes together to make beautiful music. This is a perfect analogy. And in an orchestra, the final music depends on the skill and coordination of the musicians. The same is true in surgery. This is why the proper surgeon and the proper surgical team are so critical.

WHAT SHOULD I LOOK FOR IN A FACILITY?

In addition to finding the right surgeon and surgical team, you want to assure that you are being treated in an excellent facility and will receive excellent follow up care. The facility should be well equipped for the treatment you need and have a great track record of positive results. Consider the devices they use, their facilities, success rates, complication rates, infection control, and more.

At our facility, we are able to control the infection rate in a way that many hospitals cannot. Because we only perform surgery on an elective basis, many sources of infection are excluded or reduced. In addition, although Germany enjoys a very low MRSA infection rate when compared to the U.S. and Canada, we have had zero cases of MRSA due to the screening measures in place. Infection rates are carefully monitored by the German government and can be verified through them.

Remember, a good surgical result does not end with the surgery. For the best possible outcome, a patient must have proper post-operative care. Such care includes not just medications and infection control but also can include physical therapy, nutrition, massage, and much more. Again, even the most skillfully-performed surgery, performed by the most-skilled surgeon, can go awry without proper care afterwards. Sadly, due to financial pressures, many hospitals and surgical centers force patients to leave the facility long before they should. This is an unfortunate reality in many medical systems. We are fortunate in our circumstances. Because of the nature of our relationship with the hospital, a patient can stay for many days after surgery. In fact, the typical ADR patient stays at the hospital for 4-6 days after surgery. They are then transferred to a luxurious hotel surrounded by a beautiful park, where they can recuperate further, all with the assistance of careful monitoring, physical therapy, and massage.

Remember, a good surgical result does not end with the surgery.

Explore the follow-up care procedures and protocols as part of your decision making. Make sure you are comfortable with the type and duration of care post-op.

You should also seek testimonials from past patients. More in-depth case studies are particularly beneficial. While one person's result does not predict the next person's result, you can learn a great deal from reading or watching stories from past patients. If you would like to see an example of the types of case studies you might consider, visit http://www.enande.com.

If possible, explore referrals from patients who have undergone treatment by the same surgeon, team and facility. Nothing beats personal contact, and nothing replaces the ability to ask questions.

Whatever you do, get your questions answered! Your provider should be able to answer your questions clearly and to your satisfaction. The proper and accurate exchange of information between the patient and surgeon or team is one of the best indicators of success.

CAN DISC REPLACEMENT BE UNDONE IF NEEDED?

One question we receive periodically is whether a disc replacement surgery can be "undone." This depends on the hardware used and the amount of time that has elapsed since surgery. In the weeks following surgery, the vertebrae above and below the artificial disc hardware are fusing to the hardware itself. This is exactly what is supposed to occur. Over time, the vertebra and the hardware essentially "become one." This is ideal since this keeps the disc in place so it can properly function for the rest of the patient's life.

If, for some reason, a patient decided to have the procedure reversed, this must occur within a very limited window following surgery *if the hardware is to be removed.* If the hardware is removed, a traditional fusion can still be performed.

However, if the hardware and the surrounding vertebra have mated and joined permanently, then removal of the hardware may not be appropriate. In this circumstance, traditional fusion can still be done. The disc hardware is simply left in place. In fact, we had one patient who developed severe spondylolisthesis six months after surgery. We fused the level with the disc in place, and the patient did very well afterward.

While the question of potentially reversing a disc replacement is an interesting one, it is largely academic. There is very rarely, if ever, a need to remove or attempt to reverse this procedure. For the more than four thousand patients I have treated with disc replacement, we have only had to go back and remove a disc or place a fusion around an artificial disc fewer than five times. This occurred in very few instances with early disc hardware. After having placed thousands of M6 devices, we have only ever removed discs post initial implantation on a few occasions. These were never due to a failing of the disc but due to a low grade infection later in life, where bacteria entered the body through a kidney infection or a severe oral infection and then settled on the prosthetic. As a result, the device had to be removed.

HOW LONG WILL AN ARTIFICIAL DISC LAST?

Most artificial disc implants are engineered to last for a very long time. The protocol for FDA certification in the U.S. requires the device to last for at least ten million cycles. For example, the ProDisc-C (Cervical) has been tested to ten million cycles (Synthes, 2011). The M6 device has been tested to more than 30 million cycles, after which the disc was still completely functional and within normal limits of motion and function. This means the M6 implant is expected to last for 60-75 years *before* suffering significant wear. Incidentally, this is far more durable than human discs, most of which begin to deteriorate after only 20-30 years of life.

One way devices of this nature are tested is to check the amount of wear on the device and particularly the amount of debris that wears off such a device per 1 million cycles. Testing is performed in a very closely monitored environment that is meant to resemble the human body in regards to temperature, the surrounding fluids, and the load or pressure on the disc.

Unlike some other joint implants, where we can predict that another replacement or resection will be needed in 10-20 years, a quality artificial disc should last a lifetime.

If you undergo disc replacement, you should never need to have that disc replaced in normal circumstances. Unlike some other joint implants, where we can predict that another replacement or resection will be needed in 10-20 years, a quality artificial disc should last a lifetime. Given the construction materials and techniques, modern disc implants should never need to be replaced or resected.

WHAT COMPLICATIONS CAN ARISE FROM DISC REPLACEMENT SURGERY?

There are risks associated with any surgery, and disc replacement is no different. The majority of complications associated with disc replacement surgery are not actually related to disc replacement. They arise from the approach (the procedure needed to access the disc) and suture/wound care.

INFECTION

Any surgery of this nature is subject to potential infection, both during the surgery and at the suture site after surgery. Surgeons go to great lengths to minimize the chance for such infection. Strict sterilization procedures are observed in and around the surgical suite. As such, the chance for infection is very low. Actual infection rates will vary from facility to facility and also from country to country. For instance, MRSA infection rates in the U.S. are higher than most of the world and roughly 2.5 times higher than in Germany (CDDEP, 2016).

Fortunately, MRSA infection rates have been falling. Nonetheless, there is always potential for infection in any surgery, regardless of location, facility, or surgeon. You should inquire about infection rates with any surgeon or facility you are considering. Our surgical facility actually has a ZERO percent infection rate for MRSA. This is because of extensive screening procedures as well as infection control in the hospital. Our overall infection rate is 1.8%, none of which is related to MRSA.

HEMATOMA

One potential complication that can occur primarily with cervical disc replacement is hematoma. In simple terms, this is when blood collects outside the blood vessels and places pressure on nerves and other structures. This can result in numbness and other symptoms. This is usually temporary in nature. hematoma can also result in more serious problems. As a result, your surgical team will carefully monitor your condition after surgery.

BLOOD LOSS

Blood loss is always a concern with any major surgery. Depending on the approach used and the type of procedure to be performed, this can be a significant concern. Fortunately, disc replacement surgery, when performed with the retro-peritoneal approach and by an experienced surgical team, is usually associated with very little blood loss. Furthermore, our team employs the Cell-Saver, a device which allows the surgical team to collect the patient's blood during surgery and then later use the patient's blood for replenishment rather than using a transfusion from a blood bank. This device is always present at our surgical table but is almost never needed for ADR because of minimal blood loss. While it was regularly used for prior implants and is still used for fusion and hybrid intervention, we found after implanting the first 50 or so M6 devices that this was not needed because the patients lost so little blood. We keep detailed records of the need for transfusions of any kind. Our overall transfusion rate in the hospital is 3% *across all procedures* and is almost non-existent for disc replacement. Ask your surgeon about his or her transfusion rate in general and for disc replacement specifically. He or she should be able to give you an objective answer.

APPROACH-RELATED COMPLICATIONS

Approach-related complications are the most common type of complication in disc replacement. These can occur as the surgeon cuts through or moves around tissues, blood vessels, nerves, and other structures. The likelihood of such complications increases in relation to the type of approach performed and the frequency with which the surgeon performs this approach; the less frequently a surgeon performs the approach, the more often complications can arise. This is one of the reasons you need to make sure your surgeon performs disc replacements on a very frequent basis. My surgical team performs multiple disc replacement procedures every week, and this makes us efficient and experienced at what we do. It also means we have very low complication rates.

The type of approach is important too. For lumbar disc replacement, we use a *retro*-peritoneal approach, which means we go around and behind the peritoneal cavity. In my experience, this is the safest method of accessing the lumbar spine. Not all surgeons are adept at this approach and so may use a trans-peritoneal approach instead, meaning they go *through* the peritoneum. My research has revealed that this has as much as a 15% complication rate related to the development of adhesions at the surgical site, in addition to other potential complications. Such increased complications include retrograde ejaculation as well as changes that can result in a painful and dry vagina. Ultimately, the trans-peritoneal approach has an increased risk for infertility too.

For this reason, if you need lumbar disc replacement, I highly recommend that you discuss the approach with any potential surgeon to make sure a *retro-*peritoneal approach is used.

PARALYSIS

As with any spinal surgery, there is a very slight chance of paralysis. This is extremely rare. When it does occur, it is usually temporary. In my personal practice, we have had zero instances of paralysis in lumbar disc replacement. The same hold true for cases of pure disc replacement in the cervical spine. We have had three instances of paralysis in cervical patients who were receiving a hybrid intervention involving disc replacement along with fusion. All were related to post-surgical hematoma (a solid swelling of clotted blood) pressing against or located in the spinal cord. There was no direct injury to the spinal cord caused by the surgeon.

In one of these instances, we were able to relieve the pressure on the spinal cord, and the patient improved. In a second, the patient, who had significant neurological deficits due to myelopathy before surgery, worsened after surgery despite the fact that we were able to relieve the pressure with a follow-up surgery. Unfortunately, in the third case, we were unable alleviate the hematoma. For this reason, we always advise patients of the possibility of permanent paralysis, but this has occurred precisely twice in the more than 4000 patients we have treated with ADR. In all of these cases, the complications arose *not* as a result of disc replacement but in association with the fusion portion of a hybrid intervention.

It should also be noted that *when* you have surgery can have an impact on your results. Many patients seeking spinal surgery suffer from myelopathy, neurologic deficits resulting from injury to the spinal cord. This refers not just to pain but also numbness, tingling, decreased reflexes, partial paralysis, etc. that arise from impingement of the spinal cord by the disc, part of a vertebrae, or other body. Myelopathy typically gets worse over time, and the long-term effects increase over time. While disc replacement may be able to relieve pressure on the spinal cord, the results of myelopathy may linger for a long time, especially if this myelopathy existed for a long time prior to surgery.   For this reason, getting your myelopathy addressed in a timely manner is critical.

NERVE/SENSORY CHANGES

Another potential complication involves changes in sensation or feelings of numbness. This has occurred in six or seven of our disc replacement patients and was temporary for roughly half of these instances. This equates to roughly a 0.16% rate, or roughly 1 out of every 615 patients. In each of these cases, the complication involves sensation, numbness or tingling but did not involve function, motion, or control.

OTHER COMPLICATIONS

There are other potential complications that can occur with disc replacement, and with any surgery. You should discuss these complications with your surgeon and inquire about their experience with these complications. You should also feel free to ask your surgeon what steps he or she takes to minimize the chance of such complications.   While there is no such thing as a risk-free surgery, selecting the proper surgeon and surgical team can go a long way toward minimizing your risks.

We carefully track complication rates at our facility. In rough terms, here are our results: Our overall complication rate, including all possible complications, is approximately 2%. This incredibly low rate of complication is due to a combination of factors: proper diagnosis, skill of the surgeon and surgical team, frequency with which procedures are performed, top-notch facility, proper follow-up care, and more. The vast majority (about 90%) of the complications that do arise involve superficial wound-healing problems. Another 5% (of the 2%!) consists of distraction pain of more than four weeks in duration. Subsidence or migration of the disc, neurologic complications, and other factors each comprise less than 1% (of the 2%) individually.

While there is no such thing as a risk-free surgery, selecting the proper surgeon and surgical team can go a long way toward minimizing your risks.

You should feel comfortable asking your surgeon and facility for their complication rate. If they seem unable (or unwilling) to provide to you this information, you may wish to consider another provider.

SHOULD I PUT OFF DISC REPLACEMENT AS LONG AS POSSIBLE?

Many people who have been told they should have spinal fusion have also been told they should put such fusion off as long as possible. It is not uncommon for patients to be told they should simply live with their pain until they cannot stand it any longer, and *then* get fusion. This has come about because we know, over time, spinal fusion at one level will cause increased stress and degeneration at adjacent levels. Eventually, those adjacent levels may require fusion. Therefore, there are disadvantages to having fusion early rather than late.

The same discussion occurs around knee and hip replacements, where such implants have a limited lifespan before they may have to be resected or redone.

Fortunately, this problem does not exist for most artificial disc devices. Because of the incredible durability of the implants, we know that a single implant will last a patient for the rest of his or her life. As a result, there is no advantage to putting off disc replacement in most circumstances. There are limited situations where a surgeon may want to delay surgery to get other conditions and factors under control, but there is otherwise no advantage to putting off surgery. On the contrary, there *are* some instances where delay can be problematic, particularly if the delay allows the underlying disease to progress so far that it damages the integrity of the vertebrae. In addition, the longer the nerves are impinged often means that recovery may be more difficult, or more limited. And, the longer you wait for surgery, the more deconditioned your muscles and other structures may become. Sadly, poor conditioning can cause a mediocre or poor result from an otherwise excellent surgery. For these reasons, if you are a candidate for surgery, consider getting it done as soon as reasonable. At the very least, explore your options now and have a frank discussion with your surgeon about the pros and cons of waiting for surgery. You may find that surgery in the near future may serve you better.

WHAT KIND OF REHABILITATION IS RECOMMENDED FOLLOWING DISC REPLACEMENT?

The nature of rehabilitation following spinal surgery varies greatly around the world. In North America, many spinal surgery patients are sent home one to two days after surgery, largely for financial reasons. The cost of a hospital stay is simply so extreme that there is great pressure on the surgeon to get patients out of the hospital at the first opportunity. Once patients are transferred home, they often receive little to no monitoring or treatment, sometimes receiving their first follow-up care weeks (and even months) after their surgery.

This is quite different in other portions of the world. At our facilities, patients are allowed to remain in the hospital for 4-10 days depending on their surgery. Although disc replacement patients can usually stand and walk on their own the day following surgery, we prefer to allow them to recuperate in an environment that is both safe and comfortable. While in the hospital, we can provide appropriate pain control, physical therapy and even massage, all very effective treatment methods. Such post-surgical care is critical given the changes that occur with disc replacement. Since the discs have restored the long-compromised spacing between the vertebrae, there is a certain amount of stretching of the surrounding muscles and soft tissue. Physical therapy, stretching, massage, and heat packs are excellent modalities, so we provide these to the patient immediately and repeatedly during recovery in our hospitals.

Even after the hospital stay, our patients are transferred to an exclusive hotel surrounded by a very large park, a perfect setting for rest and recovery. We send our physical therapist and a masseur to the hotel to provide additional therapy and massage. We continue to monitor the patients there until they reach nearly two weeks post surgery, at which time they are seen for another in-depth examination.

Sadly, this level of care is difficult to provide in the U.S. and Canada, where limitations (financial and otherwise) serve to curtail the kind of rehabilitation measures that will provide the best result in the long run.

IS DISC REPLACEMENT RIGHT FOR ME?

Disc replacement is not for everyone. As you have read, not everyone is a good candidate for the procedure. Yet the truth of the matter is that most people suffering from degenerative disc disease, post-discectomy or post-discotomy syndrome, and other conditions can benefit from disc replacement in a profound and positive way. Many people who receive spinal fusions could instead have full function of the spine restored through disc replacement. And those who already have fusions in place may benefit from disc replacement if they start to have problems at adjacent levels (Adjacent Level Syndrome).

But what about you? Is this the best solution for *your* spine?

No book can accurately diagnose a medical condition, and nothing can be a substitute for sound, medical advice. While disc replacement may be a wonderful solution for you, you need to seek appropriate medical advice. I encourage you to do two things.

First, discuss disc replacement with your personal physician. Provided that he or she is familiar with your spine, input from your physician is very important. If your physician is unfamiliar with disc replacement, then give him or her a copy of this book. You can also direct your physician to www.enande.com/resources, where we have compiled studies and other resources specifically for physicians who wish to know more about the topic.

Second, I want to offer you the opportunity to have me and my team personally evaluate your condition. Our team of surgeons has performed thousands of disc replacement procedures. We know what to look for, and we know the proper indications for disc replacement or, if needed, hybrid intervention. We also have an excellent protocol for evaluating patients remotely and have been doing this for more than 10 years. Just send an email containing your full name and email address to evaluation@enande.com, and we will reply right away.

WHAT DOES ADR SURGERY COST?

The cost of disc replacement is a common concern for many patients. And with the advent of medical tourism, more and more people are researching their options as they seek out the best surgical team and the best devices from around the world. While the price of surgery should never be the primary factor in these decisions, it *is* a factor after all.

The cost of disc replacement surgery depends on numerous variables. These can include:

- Number of levels to be addressed
- Implant(s) to be used
- Type of approach and procedure
- Facility
- Surgical Team
- Length of hospital stay
- Length and nature of follow-up care

There are many more variables. Surgery and hospital costs in general vary greatly throughout the world. Surgical expenses and hospital stays in the United States, for instance, are notoriously expensive. One study showed the average hospital stay in the U.S. was 300% higher than in Germany, for instance (McMahon, 2012). In fact, physician and hospital fees in the U.S. rank at the top in study after study when compared to other developed countries.

For this reason, it is difficult to provide a clear price range for ADR surgery.

However, the cost of *not* having ADR surgery is worth discussing. I recently witnessed an online discussion where one patient explained that he had spent at least $100,000 on his back and neck so far. Even though he lives in Canada, where a certain level of care is provided without charge, he invested in

Chiropractors, Physical Therapists, Acupuncturists, and other medical and allied health professionals. He paid for medications, assistive devices, and a variety of diagnostic studies on his own. In an effort to find some way to alleviate his pain, he invested in alternative therapies, hydro aerobics, and more. He explained that he figures he has averaged at least $5000 a year in expenses for his back and neck.

He then started to count the financial cost of lost opportunities. He said he gave up $8,000 in available overtime in just the previous summer. He had to change his work duties to a sedentary position, one he only tolerates because it allows him to at least keep working. And then there are all the times he has been off work due to flare-ups, sometimes for months at a time. The money adds up quickly.

And yet, many people with severe back pain will tell you the money is the smallest part of it. The real cost is emotional and relational. This man described himself as athletic and a lover of outdoor sports. "They were my outlets," he said, "hiking, sports, walking etc...taken away from me one at a time because I would be in so much pain." He goes on to say, "All of a sudden, you're not going to see your friends because you are just 'down.' You want to, but you make excuses because it is uncomfortable to sit for a long period of time. After a while, you can't even relate to some of the good stories people are talking about (when they went for a beautiful hike and such), so you tend to avoid these things."

Like others, this man describes a cost to relationships with friends and loved ones, all because of his neck and back pain. Many people in these situations fall into some degree of depression, and that, too, causes its own problems.

Back pain costs society an enormous amount of money. The World Health Organization estimates that back pain costs the Unites States alone 100 to 200 billion dollars each year! (WHO, 2004) But those who experience back pain firsthand (and those that live and work with them) know the cost is far greater. The cost to relationships, at work and at home, can be devastating. How can we place a value on the ability of a father to support his family? Or a mother to lift her child? Simply put, we cannot. These factors, though more subjective than the money paid for medical care or the compensation lost due to time off work, are ultimately without price...or priceless.

When people discuss the cost of disc replacement surgery, these other factors need to be considered. Although ADR surgery is often far less expensive than people fear (especially when performed in Europe), the reality is that this is an *investment* and one with an incredible rate of return. This investment, naturally, needs to be weighed against the risks of surgery, but what is the value of a restored spine? Of a life without severe pain? Of a life without the constant fear of re-injury? While there can be no guaranteed outcome, our patients tell us time and time again that we have given them their lives back. And these are the words that inspire me to continue my work at the surgery table.

CASE STUDY: SANDRA LEBLANC

Single-level cervical artificial disc recipient, with surgery performed in 2012:

I am a nurse, and I work in long-term and short-term rehabilitation settings. I am also a very private person, so sharing this story is a big stretch for me.

In 2011, I injured my neck in an auto accident. Though it left me shaken and in pain, I thought it would go away. My Naturopath suggested therapy and other measures. I have always avoided medications, especially pain medications, where possible. Frankly, I have seen the long-term effects of pharmaceuticals on kidneys, and I have seen too many people addicted to opiate pain killers. So pain meds weren't really an option for me.

Over time, I started to get worse. I was in horrible pain. In fact, it got so bad I could not turn my neck at all. And then I lost most of the use of my left arm! So I sought other solutions, from an Orthopaedic surgeon. After testing and imaging, he told me I needed a 2-level cervical fusion. I was crushed. I have encountered plenty of people in my life who have undergone fusions, and it just seems that every single one is worse after the surgery.

CASE STUDY: SANDRA LEBLANC (CONT.)

I sought a second opinion, and a third. Each doctor told me the same thing: 2-level cervical fusion.

This was a tough time for me. I was still working. As a single mother, there was no way I could afford to take time off from work or go on disability. So I kept working through the pain, at least as well as a could with an immobile neck and without pain meds.

At the same time, I started to research other options. There just had to be a solution better than a fusion. I knew about Adjacent Level Syndrome, where a fusion at one level often later causes the need for a fusion at adjacent levels. This was not for me.

During this time, I learned about Artificial Disc Replacement. I was doing research on the internet almost every day after work when I discovered this alternative to fusion. I was pretty skeptical at first. When I learned I might need to travel to another county to do it, I was even more concerned.

I am a nurse; I work in the U.S. medical system. To depart the U.S. and seek care abroad is a pretty foreign idea to me, or at least it was at the time.

So I kept doing research, exhaustive research. And all of it kept pointing me to disc replacement. The more I researched disc replacement, the more I realized that I needed to be evaluated by Dr. Ritter-Lang and the surgical team at Enande. The strange thing is this: after I sent my tests and films to Enande, Dr. Ritter-Lang informed me that I didn't need treatment at two levels after all. Rather than getting a 2-level fusion here, I really only needed a single artificial disc.

As great as this news was, I was still struggling. I discovered that my insurance was more than happy to pay for a 2-level fusion here, but they wouldn't pay for a single-level disc replacement in Germany, even though the surgery would be much less expensive for them...and better for me. Given the financial concern, I was really torn. In the midst of my dilemma, my Chiropractor asked me a life-changing question.

She said, "Sandra, if you had all the money in the world, what would you do?"

"I would go to Germany!" I said, without hesitation.

That is when it all became clear for me. Money was in no way more important than my spine.

CASE STUDY: SANDRA LEBLANC (CONT.)

And no amount of help from the insurance company was worth going through fusion, and then maybe another and another.

November 2, 2012. That's the day I underwent cervical Artificial Disc Replacement. The surgical team at Enande replaced the disc at C5-6 with the M6 device from Spinal Kinetics. And rather than being given a handful of Percocet and getting rushed out of the hospital within 24 hours of surgery here in the States, they allowed me to rest in the ICU for 24 hours with a morphine drip to eliminate pain. And then they moved me to my very spacious room to begin my rehabilitation. There was no suffering at all. And the staff was very friendly and helpful. There was no problem with a language barrier, and I really appreciated the on-site physical therapy and massage, something I would never have received back home.

As a nurse, I found the level of care to be very good. Whenever I needed something, they came right away. Most places here in the States don't handle just Orthopaedics. Having that facility there in Germany is a great advantage because the nurses and staff are dealing with the same issues over and over. This allows them to focus on orthopedic problems and develop expertise.

I waited 12 weeks after surgery to return to work, mainly because Dr. Ritter-Lang told me not to lift more than 20 lbs until 3 months had passed. But when I came back to work, it was full duty, lifting patients at times, moving and rotating them when needed, etc.

It has been about four years since my disc replacement, and I feel very good. I have complete motion of my neck, and I experience no pain at all. None! This is a far cry from my completely immobile (and painful) neck before surgery. As it is, I may just choose to work into my 80s!

I couldn't be happier with my surgery with Enande and the surgical team. I have referred others for disc replacement as well. In fact, I keep Enande's contact info in my purse at all times, and I am always giving it out. The truth is, not everyone will research this like I did (and I researched this extensively!). Spine surgery is a scary thing to do, and going to another country for surgery is even more scary. But I know I made the correct decision for my spine...and my life.

Sandra Leblanc, USA

5

THE FUTURE OF FUSION ALTERNATIVES

WHAT DOES THE FUTURE HOLD?

THE FUTURE OF artificial disc replacement and fusion alternatives in general is very exciting. After the decades of early experimentation with disc implants in the 60s, 70s and 80s, we have really reached the "golden age" of disc replacement. The 90s saw (for some of the world anyway) the general establishment of disc replacement as a viable alternative to spinal fusion, and the last 15 years have allowed the perfection of the surgical procedures and the development of ideal hardware solutions.

This is an incredible time. Artificial disc replacement has moved far beyond the experimental stage and is now recognized as an established and highly successful method for treating a variety of spinal conditions. While disc replacement is still limited in application in the U.S. and Canada, it is now considered the preferred and state-of-the-art alternative to spinal fusion in most of the developed world. Even in the U.S. and Canada, disc replacement is starting to take hold, though it may be many years before U.S. and Canadian surgeons (and their teams) develop the level of experience that can be found elsewhere.

With the increased utilization of disc replacement, hybrid solutions involving disc replacement with fusion are now being used more frequently to treat conditions where disc replacement alone is not appropriate. This means more people are receiving the benefits of disc replacement to the greatest extent possible, and more people are returning to fully-functional lives.

The future of fusion alternatives is very promising. Building on the work that has been done, there will certainly be new implants introduced. While I find this exciting, I know that any improvements from new implants will be very incremental in nature. The current state-of-the-art devices are extremely solid and reliable, and it is difficult to imagine any dramatic improvement. The greatest likelihood of change will come in the devices and procedures approved in North America, which is sadly lagging the rest of the developed world in this area. In the next five to ten years, we will likely see some of the best devices used in the rest of the world finally coming to use in the U.S. and Canada. Maybe someday we will see more multi-level disc replacement options approved by the FDA. Even then, the depth of experience in providing multi-level ADR may be lacking. Until then, patients desiring the best devices, multi-level options, and hybrid solutions may continue to look to Europe.

We now have decades of experience with modern implants and procedures, and the results are extremely favorable. After more than 4,000 successful disc replacement surgeries (and over 6,500 implanted devices) performed by myself and my team, I have had a chance to witness incredible recoveries, including patients who have returned to professional horseback riding, Iron Man triathlons, competitive volleyball, professional golf and much, much more. As exciting as these stories are, the most important stories are far more poignant: the man who can return to work and support his family; the woman who can walk after being told she would be confined to a wheelchair; the young father whose back pain restricted him to living on the floor but who now can live a normal life and be the dad he always wanted to be. These are the stories that make me so excited about what we do.

The future will be even better. More and more people will get to benefit from disc replacement. And we will hear more and more success stories and see more lives changed. It is an honor to have been part of the history and development of disc replacement, and it will be a greater honor as we move forward into its future.

Karsten Ritter-Lang, M.D.

REFERENCES

CDDEP (2016, November 21). *MRSA infection rates by country.* Retrieved from Center for Disease Dynamics, Economics & Policy: http://www.cddep.org/tool/mrsa_infection_rates_countr y

FDA (2004, October 26). *2004 Device Approvals.* Retrieved from U.S. Food & Drug Administration: http://www.fda.gov/medicaldevices/productsandmedical procedures/deviceapprovalsandclearances/recently-approveddevices/ucm080693.htm

FDA (2006, August 14). *2006 Device Approvals.* Retrieved from U.S. Food & Drug Administration: http://www.fda.gov/medicaldevices/productsandmedical procedures/deviceapprovalsandclearances/recently-approveddevices/ucm077620.htm

FDA (2007). *2007 Device Approvals.* Retrieved from U.S. Food & Drug Administration: http://www.fda.gov/MedicalDevices/ProductsandMedical Procedures/DeviceApprovalsandClearances/Recently-ApprovedDevices/ucm073314.htm

FDA (2007, July 17). *FDA Approves First of a Kind Medical Device to Treat Cervical Degenerative Disc Disease.* Retrieved from FDA News Release: http://www.fda.gov/newsevents/newsroom/pressannoun cements/2007/ucm108950.htm

FDA (2016, November 21). *Premarket Approval (PMA).* Retrieved from U.S. Food & Drug Administration: https://www.accessdata.fda.gov/scripts/cdrh/cfdocs/cfp ma/pma.cfm

Ironman Triathlon (2016, November 23). Retrieved from Wikipedia: https://en.wikipedia.org/wiki/Ironman_Triathlon

Lee, J. (2014, March 22). *Rethinking Spine Care.* Retrieved from Modern Healthcare: http://www.modernhealthcare.com/article/20140322/MA GAZINE/303229985

McMahon, P. (2012, March 6). *Worldwide price survey puts U.S. medical, hospital costs at top.* Retrieved from Los Angeles

Times:
http://articles.latimes.com/2012/mar/06/business/la-fi-mo-u.s.-medical-prices-high-20120306

Moenning, J., Bussard, D., Lapp, T., & Garrison, B. (1995). Average blood loss and the risk of requiring perioperative blood transfusion in 506 orthognathic surgical procedures. *Journal of Oral and Maxillofacial Surgery, 53*(8), 880-883. Retrieved from PubMed: https://www.ncbi.nlm.nih.gov/pubmed/7629615

National Council for Osteopathic Research (2012). *Oswestry Disability Index (ODI).* Retrieved from National Councisl for Osteopathic   Research: http://www.ncor.org.uk/wp-content/uploads/2012/12/Oswestry-Disability-questionnairev2.pdf

Nguyen, T., Randolph, D., Talmage, J., Succop, P., & Travis, R. (2011, February 15). Long-term outcomes of lumbar fusion among workers' compensation subjects: a historical cohort study. *Spine, 36*(4), 320-321. Retrieved from Pub Med: https://www.ncbi.nlm.nih.gov/pubmed/20736894

Oswestry Disability Index (2016). Retrieved from Wikipedia: https://en.wikipedia.org/wiki/Oswestry_Disability_Index

Patients Beyond Borders. (2016, August 6). *Medical Tourism Statistics & Facts.* Retrieved from Patients Beyond Borders: http://www.patientsbeyondborders.com/medical-tourism-statistics-facts

Sears, W., Sergides, I., Kazemi, N., Smith, M., White, G., & Osburg, B. (2011). Incidence and prevalence of surgery at segments adjacent to a previous posterior lumbar arthrodesis. *Spine, 11*(1), 11-20. Retrieved from ncbi.nlm.nih.gov/pubmed

Siepe, C. J., Mayer, H. M., Wiechert, K., & Korge, A. (2006). Clinical Results of total Lumbar Disc Replacement With ProDisc II: three-Year Results for Different Indications. *Spine, 31*(17), 1923-1932. Retrieved from http://www.medscape.com/viewarticle/542479_3

Spinal Kinetics (2009, February 18). *Spinal Kinetics Implants First M6-L Artificial Lumbar Disk.* Retrieved from Spinal Kinetics: spinalkinetics.com/wp-content/themes/sk/pdf/Spinal-Kinetics-PR-021809.pdf

Synthes (2011, August). *ProDisc-C Total Disc Replacement.* Retrieved from Synthes:

http://www.synthes.com/sites/NA/NAContent/Docs/Prod
uct%20Support%20Materials/PDF-
PowerPoints/SPINE/ProDisc-C_Product_info.pdf

WHO (2004). *Priority diseases and reasons for inclusion.* Retrieved
from World Health Organization:
http://www.who.int/medicines/areas/priority_medicines/
Ch6_24LBP.pdf

Whoriskey, P., & Keating, D. (2013, October 27). *Spinal Fusions
Serve as Case Study for Debate Over When Certain Surgeries
are Necessary.* Retrieved from Washington Post:
http://www.washingtonpost.com/business/economy/spin
al-fusions-serve-as-case-study-for-debate-over-when-
certain-surgeries-are-necessary/2013/10/27/5f015efa-
25ff-11e3-b3e9-d97fb087acd6_story.html

ABOUT THE AUTHORS

DR. KARSTEN RITTER-LANG

Spinal Surgeon, Head of Spinal Surgery

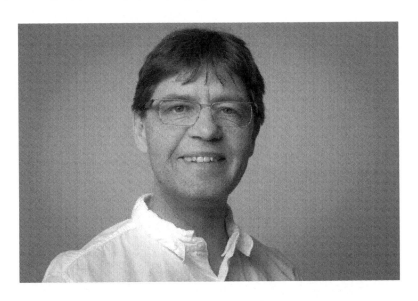

Dr. Ritter-Lang began his career in Berlin at the Charite University Hospital, the birthplace of disc replacement. He is now the Head of the Spinal Surgery Department at two hospitals and continues in private practice.

Following his medical studies at The Humboldt University in Berlin, Dr. Ritter-Lang worked and taught at the Charite University Hospital, widely recognized as the birthplace of the first effective artificial disc. Dr. Ritter-Lang has been a specialist in the field of intervertebral disc prosthetics, especially in the field of abdominal approach surgery, for over 20 years. He has performed approximately 10,000 surgeries, over 4,000 of which have involved disc replacement. He has also performed several thousand fusions and hundreds of hybrid interventions in his ongoing career.

Dr. Ritter-Lang is one of the most internationally-respected speakers regarding spinal surgery and disc replacement. His participation in the ongoing development of intervertebral disc prosthetics technology, prototypes, and implants makes him a valuable resource for other spine surgeons, who travel from around the world to observe and model his surgical techniques. He has assembled an elite surgical team that specializes in disc replacement and hybrid intervention, and patients frequently seek his care because of his and his team's experience and the increased number of options his team can provide. Dr. Ritter-Lang is one of the most experienced disc replacement surgeons in the world, and he has dedicated his career to this sub-specialty.

DR. JAN SPILLER

Orthopedic Surgeon, Chief Surgeon

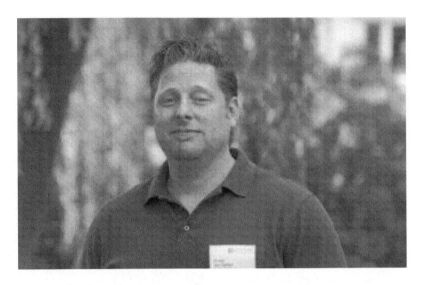

Dr. Spiller studied at Georg August University Göttingen and completed his doctoral thesis on Surgical Therapies of Specific and Unspecific Spondylitis. He began his specialized orthopedic training under Dr. Ritter-Lang and Dr. Zechel in 2004 and earned an additional degree in Chiropractic Therapy and Sports Medicine in 2008. Dr. Spiller also earned a specialization in Trauma Surgery at Klinikum Bremen Mitte under Prof. Dr. Hahn. He became Senior Surgeon at Stenum Hospital in 2010. He currently is the Chief Surgeon at Stenum Hospital, specializing in orthopedic surgery, spinal surgery, and joint surgery.

COMPLIMENTARY EVALUATION

YOU MAY ALREADY know you want to explore disc replacement or hybrid interventions, also sometimes referred to as hybrid surgery. Or you may know you want a second opinion from me and my highly experienced surgical team. If so, I want to extend to you the opportunity for an in-depth, comprehensive and *complimentary* evaluation. Simply email your full name and email address to evaluation@enande.com, and we will respond right away.

PASS IT ALONG!

DO YOU KNOW someone else who suffers from severe back or neck pain? Do you know someone else who needs to "get their back back?"

If so, please consider passing this book along. Everybody deserves to be educated about their options for spinal care. The more people know about disc replacement, the more people can enjoy the freedom that comes with it. Pass this book along to a friend, coworker, or loved one. They will thank you for it!

Made in the USA
San Bernardino, CA
28 March 2017